THE
COMPLETE

LYMPHEDEMA

MANAGEMENT AND
NUTRITION GUIDE

THE
COMPLETE

LYMPHEDEMA

MANAGEMENT AND NUTRITION GUIDE

Empowering Strategies, Supporting Recipes & Therapeutic Exercises

JEAN LAMANTIA, RD
AND **ANN DIMENNA**, PT, CDT

With foreword by EWA SZUMACHER, MD, FRCP(C), MEd

Robert
ROSE

Disclaimer

This book is a general guide only and should never be a substitute for the skill, knowledge and experience of a qualified medical professional dealing with the facts, circumstances and symptoms of a particular case.

The nutritional, medical and health information presented in this book is based on the research, training and professional experience of the authors, and is true and complete to the best of their knowledge. However, this book is intended only as an informative guide for those wishing to know more about health, nutrition and medicine; it is not intended to replace or countermand the advice given by the reader's personal physician. Because each person and situation is unique, the authors and the publisher urge the reader to check with a qualified health-care professional before using any procedure where there is a question as to its appropriateness. The authors and the publisher are not responsible for any adverse effects or consequences resulting from the use of the information in this book. It is the responsibility of the reader to consult a physician or other qualified health-care professional regarding their personal care.

This book contains references to products that may not be available everywhere. The intent of the information provided is to be helpful; however, there is no guarantee of results associated with the information provided. Use of brand names is for educational purposes only and does not imply endorsement.

The recipes in this book have been carefully tested by our kitchen and our tasters. To the best of our knowledge, they are safe and nutritious for ordinary use and users. For those people with food or other allergies, or who have special food requirements or health issues, please read the suggested contents of each recipe carefully and determine whether or not they may create a problem for you. All recipes are used at the risk of the consumer. We cannot be responsible for any hazards, loss or damage that may occur as a result of any recipe use. For those with special needs, allergies, requirements or health problems, in the event of any doubt, please contact your medical adviser prior to the use of any recipe.

At the time of publication, all URLs linked to existing websites. Robert Rose Inc. is not responsible for maintaining, and does not endorse the content of, any website or content not created by Robert Rose Inc.

Design and production: Daniella Zanchetta/PageWave Graphics Inc.
Editor: Sue Sumeraj
Copy editor: Kelly Jones
Proofreader and indexer: Gillian Watts
Images prepress preparation and color correction by Mark Veldhoven at Pixel Ink Retouching

Front cover images: Vegetarian chili © iStockphoto.com/Rudisill; Elastic bandage © iStockphoto.com/Zhekos; Tropical smoothie © iStockphoto.com/Natashamam; Fitness equipment © iStockphoto.com/Antonio Diaz
Back cover images: Orange chicken salad © iStockphoto.com/Oleg Breslavtsev; Weights/tape © iStockphoto.com/Simarik
Interior images: see page 278 for details

The publisher gratefully acknowledges the financial support of our publishing program by the Government of Canada through the Canada Book Fund.

Canada

Published by Robert Rose Inc.
120 Eglinton Avenue East, Suite 800, Toronto, Ontario, Canada M4P 1E2
Tel: (416) 322-6552 Fax: (416) 322-6936
www.robertrose.ca

Printed and bound in the USA

1 2 3 4 5 6 7 8 9 LSC 27 26 25 24 23 22 21 20 19

This book is dedicated to
people living with lymphedema.

Contents

Foreword

Lymphedema is the swelling caused by the abnormal accumulation of lymphatic fluid in the skin. It can be caused by burns, injury, surgery, radiation therapy, obesity or circulatory problems. Cancer patients are at a high risk of lymphedema following cancer treatments such as surgery and radiation.

Ann DiMenna and Jean LaMantia's book is a comprehensive guide that helps patients and health-care providers better understand lymphedema, outlining diagnostic and therapeutic approaches to control lymphedema and to prevent its complications. It is one of relatively few books that bring together all of the current knowledge and understanding of lymphedema and its pathogenesis, investigations, staging and management. Most importantly, the information is written with the patient in mind; its clear, approachable style empowers patients and their family members so they can understand the medical terminology and participate in the decision-making processes with their therapists and doctors.

This is one of relatively few books that bring together all of the current knowledge and understanding of lymphedema and its pathogenesis, investigations, staging and management.

Ann DiMenna is a certified lymphedema therapist well known for her expertise in the field of lymphedema and has been treating patients with this condition for many years, with very good results. Jean LaMantia is a registered dietitian and has focused her expertise on cancer survivorship, and she now also helps cancer survivors and others affected by lymphedema by helping to establish nutrition guidelines that support traditional methods of lymphedema management.

Together they have produced a well-structured and easy-to-understand text, and the book is illustrated with many instructional graphics, charts, diagrams and photographs that help patients understand the many different therapeutic approaches (such as bandaging, taping, exercise, and stocking and sleeve pulling) and the nutritional recommendations. These photos and images will help the reader understand and remember the important strategies Ann and Jean recommend.

The first part of the book discusses pathophysiology and the causative factors of lymphedema. It also covers lymphedema risk factors and risk-reduction techniques. Readers learn how to measure the affected limbs and chart this data for a systematic approach to measurement and follow-up.

In the second part of the book, the authors outline the different therapeutic procedures used in the treatment of lymphedema — such as manual lymphatic drainage, bandaging, pumping, taping and exercising — and describe how to use these tools properly and efficiently. The information is clearly supported by pictures and examples from Ann's practice.

The third part of the book, written by Jean LaMantia, discusses the role of nutrition and supplements in the management and prevention of lymphedema. Jean outlines dietary recommendations regarding fluid, protein, sodium, anti-inflammatory foods, fats and oils, body weight and nutritional supplements, illustrating how nutrition complements the traditional physical therapies outlined by Ann.

The fourth part of the book provides readers with meal plans and recipes that embrace the nutritional recommendations for lymphedema. The entire book is extremely well referenced and provides evidence-based information that the reader will find indispensable. Moreover, the authors include many resources and trustworthy websites that patients can use to expand their knowledge about the management of their condition, including informative websites about supplements and vitamins.

Without a doubt, the authors have created an exceptional resource about the contemporary management of lymphedema. I would highly recommend this excellent, practical and comprehensive guide to any patients at risk of development of lymphedema or to those who have already been diagnosed with this debilitating condition. This book is also dedicated to affected family members and health-care professionals treating patients with lymphedema. With evidence-based information, exquisite photographs, helpful Q&A and intelligible diagrams, this work will help patients manage their condition, possibly preventing serious complications that limit their quality of life.

— Ewa Szumacher, MD, FRCP(C), Med
Radiation Oncologist, Sunnybrook Odette
Cancer Centre, Toronto, Canada

With evidence-based information, exquisite photographs, helpful Q&A and intelligible diagrams, this work will help patients manage their condition, possibly preventing serious complications that limit their quality of life.

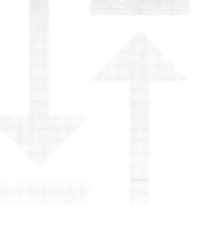

Preface

"Lymphedema is one of the most poorly understood, relatively underestimated, and least researched complications of cancer or its treatment."

— *National Cancer Institute, July 2015*

When I joined the Markham Lymphatic Centre to work with clients with lymphedema, I was shocked to find how little nutrition research has been done to help support people with this debilitating chronic disease.

It's estimated that 10 million Americans and 1 million Canadians live with lymphedema. This is a significant number of people and I am happy to do my part by using my training as a registered dietitian to research and share how nutrition can support you.

When it comes to writing a nutrition book, a person doesn't just sit down at the computer and decide what sounds like a good diet. Nutrition is a science. In fact, when writing an evidence-based nutrition book, there is actually more time spent reading research studies and fact-checking than there is writing. By collecting all of the available evidence into one book, I hope to both help those with the disease and also promote the idea that nutrition for lymphedema is an area ripe for research.

When I was first considering writing this book, I asked a lymphedema expert what he thought of the idea. His answer troubled me: "There isn't enough research to write a book about nutrition for lymphedema." But I needed to balance this with the question my clients often ask me: "Is there anything that nutrition can do to improve my lymphedema?" This books balances these seemingly opposing forces while being respectful of the research by not overpromising what nutrition can do while at the same time giving people with lymphedema some concrete nutrition strategies.

I am happy to partner with Ann DiMenna on this book. Ann is greatly admired by her clients and other professionals in the lymphedema community for her commitment to the care of individuals with lymphedema. She has grown a busy practice in Markham, Ontario, Canada, by word of mouth and she is incredibly knowledgeable and caring. She is also a trailblazer: she is one of the first lymphedema therapists that I know of to recruit a registered dietitian to her practice, as she wanted to make sure she was leaving no stone unturned in serving her clients.

It's estimated that 10 million Americans and 1 million Canadians live with lymphedema.

In our book, Ann shares all her years of experience in the physical treatment of lymphedema — and she's become quite the photographer in the process, carefully documenting what she can to help you understand and care for your lymphedema.

For my part, I summarize my thorough review of the research on nutrition for lymphedema and I have selected recipes that follow these recommendations. Because there's nothing like the voice of experience, I conducted a focus group of men and women with lymphedema of the head, neck, arm, trunk and legs to share with you their lymphedema experiences and their best advice to you. You will find their comments in the "Living with Lymphedema" sidebars throughout. We have also included "Did You Know?" boxes of supplementary information, a full glossary of terms, and references to all of the research that we cite.

I hope that this book becomes your trusted companion as you learn to care for your lymphedema. I have great compassion for you and the challenges that lymphedema brings to your life, as well as the impact on your family, work and recreation. I hope that this book supports you and makes a positive difference in your life.

Wishing you all my best,

— *Jean LaMantia, Registered Dietitian*

I hope that this book becomes your trusted companion as you learn to care for your lymphedema.

Introduction

Lymphedema is a rarely diagnosed and fairly misunderstood medical condition. Most medical schools teach little to no information regarding the lymphatic system. My first exposure to lymphedema was during a home visit as a community care physiotherapist in Toronto. I had been a physiotherapist for 2 years and didn't understand why a patient had been referred to me for shoulder exercises to improve movement when the patient's real issue was a very swollen, heavy arm. Being a very eager recent graduate, I searched for solutions to help her. I recalled a one-hour lecture I had in my second year of physiotherapy school that explained that swelling could be a possible side effect of cancer treatments. I began to search for a more appropriate therapist for her but found very few resources in her local community. I never wanted to have a referral I could not help.

This is a very underdiagnosed and misdiagnosed condition, yet it is a very common one and it affects people from all walks of life. Each lymphedema case presents its own separate challenges and requires an individual treatment plan. No two cases are alike.

This began my search for complete decongestive therapy (CDT) training and certification. I spent several months researching and training with Integrated Lymphatic Therapy here in Toronto. I looked to draw on the expertise of other physiotherapists who had treated this condition, but to my shock and dismay, I found very few within the Greater Toronto Area, let alone in the province. Having exhausted the few resources in Ontario, I headed to the United States for the National Lymphedema Network conference, learning and drawing on the expertise and research community in the U.S. I brought much of my knowledge back to Canada to help treat lymphedema patients, mostly in clients' home settings, where I saw the most difficult and complex cases — those who could not leave their homes, given how severe and painful their lymphedema condition was. Working through these complex cases is where the elements of complete decongestive therapy shine.

I have been treating lymphedema for almost 10 years, and I am reminded daily that this is a very underdiagnosed and misdiagnosed condition, yet it is a very common one and it affects people from all walks of life. I have treated cases of lymphedema as a result of obesity, cancer treatments, crush injuries from motor vehicle accidents, caesarean sections, burns, orthopedic surgeries, forceful muscle tears, severe ankle sprains, lipedema and neurological conditions — and the list goes on. The challenge I face on a daily basis is that each lymphedema case presents its own separate challenges and requires an individual treatment plan. No two cases are alike.

I strive each day to help patients living with lymphedema learn self-management strategies and try to gain control of this chronic condition. I am always amazed by the persistence, perseverance and courage patients show each and every day. It is from their strength that I feel more motivated to continue on this journey to generate and disseminate more resources, more information and more education to help everyone in the lymphedema community.

After hearing patient after patient tell me about a flare-up of swelling after a dinner party or restaurant dinner, I began my search for a dietitian who could help me piece together the link between diet and lymphedema. I first learned about Jean LaMantia several years ago when I was asked by the Lymphedema Association of Ontario to help organize a conference. I felt it was a good idea to partner with a dietitian who understood cancer and nutrition, since many people with lymphedema developed the condition following their cancer treatment. Jean has been a welcome addition to our clinic and brings a depth and breadth of nutrition knowledge, excellent problem-solving skills and a nutrition-research focus to our practice.

One day approximately 3 years ago, I received a phone call from a lymphedema patient who asked if I performed home visits; she was unable to descend the stairs outside her home because of her lymphedema symptoms. During my initial assessment, this patient told me she had suffered from lymphedema for 2 years and that it was progressively getting worse. She showed me photo albums full of vacation photos and told me that she had planned to continue traveling with her husband in her retirement. Her love of traveling the world and having amazing experiences was all on hold now because of her lymphedema. Instead of dogsledding up north or walking among the penguins, she struggled to get down the stairs. She told me she would be happy if I could help her with her swollen legs and was resigned to the fact that she might never travel again, because a doctor had informed her that air travel could cause her legs to flare up.

I treated this patient with intensive complete decongestive therapy, including manual lymphatic drainage, bandaging, skin care and exercise. Finally, after 2 months of treatment, the swelling in her legs had decreased enough that she could easily navigate stairs, outdoor activities, exercise and caring for her grandchildren. Happy with her results, she was ecstatic to be given a "new lease on life" and wanted to push the boundaries to see if she could once again travel the world — and that she did. With a lot of knowledge, self–manual lymphatic drainage and self-bandaging for her flights, she continued to travel. She is a prime example of how important self-management strategies are to every treatment plan. And although your goals may be different, everyone can benefit from having a toolbox full of self-management techniques.

Although your goals may be different, everyone can benefit from having a toolbox full of self-management techniques.

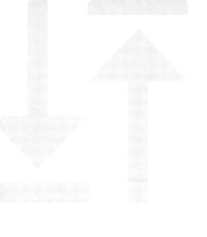

When I was asked to co-author this book with Jean, I was excited about producing an all-inclusive management guide to help people living with lymphedema. It is so important for lymphedema patients to learn self-management strategies as part of their overall treatment plan. I believe that the best outcomes in treatment materialize when patients learn self-management strategies and work with a therapist who provides complete decongestive therapy and all its components — the results are simply amazing. I always say: "What you put in, you get out." The intention of this book is not to replace the advice of your certified lymphedema therapist or medical team, but to help you understand lymphedema, learn prevention tactics and self-manage your lymphedema during the maintenance phase. Not all strategies presented in the book will work for you, so it is always best to consult with a CDT therapist before beginning.

My hope is that you will take advantage of all the valuable information in this book, information that is supported by unbiased high-quality scientific research. Throughout the book, you will see references such as "In 2002, Box and colleagues showed that …" In this example, we are referring to a study that was published in 2002 by a group of researchers, the first of whom has the last name Box. You can read more about all the referenced research in the References, page 259. This book also contains references to specific products and brand names. Their inclusion here does not imply endorsement; rather, I included them as examples only.

You can incorporate the management strategies, nutritional findings and recipes into your daily plan and gain more control over your lymphedema. Many of the patients in my clinical practice have shared with me strategies that work for them, and it is my hope that these strategies will also help you cope with this condition. It is with knowledge, skill, perseverance and determination that you will gain control of this condition and live well with lymphedema.

All the best,

— *Ann DiMenna, PT, CDT*

> *The best outcomes in treatment materialize when patients learn self-management strategies and work with a therapist who provides complete decongestive therapy and all its components — the results are simply amazing.*

PART 1
Understanding Lymphedema

CHAPTER 1

The Lymphatic System and Lymphedema

To understand lymphedema and why it develops, you must first understand how your lymphatic system is designed, how it works and its purpose. This chapter of the book is designed as a question-and-answer section to clearly explain how the lymphatic system works and how lymphedema develops.

How does fluid move through our bodies?

The circulation of fluids throughout the body is done via arteries, veins and lymphatic vessels. These three different vessels are all part of one system called the vascular system (also called the cardiovascular system or circulatory system).

   The arteries are the first part of the circulatory system, delivering and distributing the blood from your heart to your body's organs and tissues; the arteries transport oxygen and nutrients in the blood. The farther the arteries get from the heart, the smaller they become. The smallest arteries are called arterioles. The arterioles connect to capillaries, and these connect to small veins called venules. These grow in circumference until they become veins.

   The veins are the second part of the circulatory system, carrying the deoxygenated blood back to the heart and then on to the lungs to be reoxygenated. The volume of blood that enters the veins is estimated to be between 80% and 90% of the volume from the arteries. What happens to the other 10% to 20% of the fluid from the blood? It leaks out of the capillaries. That's where the lymphatic system comes in to help.

What is the lymphatic system?

The lymphatic system is responsible for maintaining your body's fluid balance by taking up that 10% to 20% of fluid that has leaked out of the blood capillaries, kind of like a catch basin. Without this system, that fluid would pool and swelling would be the result. Once the fluid has been absorbed, it is transported through the lymphatic vessels and delivered back to the heart to re-enter the blood vessels.

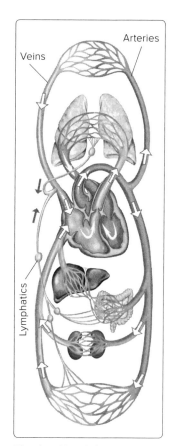

Veins

Arteries

Lymphatics

Blood and lymph fluid circulation to the body's major organs and tissues

How much lymphatic fluid does my body circulate in a day?

The volume of lymphatic fluid that circulates throughout your body changes — typically between 1 and 4 quarts (1 and 4 L) per day. This volume is dependent on a number of factors, including:

- **Activity level:** If you're very active, more blood is circulated, more fluid leaks from the capillaries and lymph accumulates.
- **Temperature:** On hot days, the body circulates more blood to the extremities to help cool you off, and more blood circulated translates into more lymph fluid.
- **Meals:** The size and number of meals per day affect the amount of lymphatic fluid in your body (lymphatic fluid increases after eating, especially fatty meals).

You can read more about this in Chapter 11: Lymphatics and the Digestion of Dietary Fats, page 142.

What is lymphatic fluid composed of?

When fluid first enters the lymphatic system, it is very similar to blood plasma. It is composed of mostly water, but it also contains protein, dead cells, bacteria and viruses; it has a clear or yellowish consistency. As the fluid moves from the lymph capillaries into the larger lymph vessels, it is mixed with more protein, long-chain fatty acids, white blood cells and cellular debris, and it becomes milky in appearance. Although it changes in consistency from the time it is first picked up by the lymphatic capillaries until it reaches the large lymphatic trunks, it is called lymph throughout.

What are the lymph nodes and where are they located?

The human body contains between 600 and 700 lymph nodes and they are dispersed throughout the body. They are grouped together in chains. Major lymph node basins are found in the armpit and in the groin. There are between 150 and 200 lymph nodes in the neck, and there is an extensive network of nodes in the abdomen, around all of the organs. The size of nodes can vary in adults and ranges from 0.08 to 1.18 inches (0.2 to 3.0 cm). They can be round, oval, spindle-like or kidney-shaped, and different-shaped nodes are found in different areas of the body.

The human body contains between 600 and 700 lymph nodes and they are dispersed throughout the body. They are grouped together in chains.

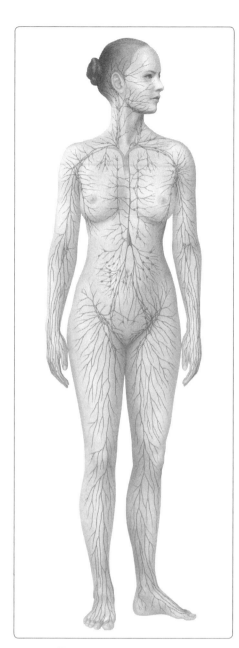

The lymphatic vessel system

What are the components of the lymphatic vessel system?

The lymphatic vessel system is composed of lymph capillaries, pre-collectors, lymph collectors and lymphatic trunks (listed in order of smallest to largest). These vessels also travel through lymph nodes and become progressively larger until they empty into the subclavian veins, thereby returning fluid back to the blood.

- **Lymph capillaries** are also called initial lymphatics and pre-lymphatics; in the digestive system, they are called lacteals and their function is different. Lymph capillaries are responsible for picking up fluid that has leaked from the blood capillaries into the spaces around cells (the interstitial spaces). The lymph capillaries do not use valves to move the fluid. The fluid flows in response to a pressure gradient, from the high pressure in the interstitial spaces into the low-pressure lymph capillaries.

- **Pre-collectors** take fluid from the small lymph capillaries and move it to larger vessels.

- **Lymph collectors** are larger vessels, and they have valves that move the fluid toward the nodes and heart.

- **Lymphatic trunks** carry the fluid back to the heart from the legs, lower body and genitals. There are two trunks — a left trunk and a right trunk — and these merge into the largest lymph trunk in the body, known as the thoracic duct. This duct transfers all lymph from the lower body and abdomen back to the heart, where it joins the blood.

How does lymphatic fluid move through the lymphatic system?

The lymph vessels are parallel to and travel with the veins, arteries and nerves throughout the entire body. The three circulatory vessels in the skin (venules, arterioles and lymphatic capillaries) are woven together like a basket weave. Unlike the blood vascular system, which begins at the heart with the largest vessels (arteries), the lymphatic system begins with its smallest vessels — lymph capillaries. The lymph capillaries take up the 10% to 20% of fluid that has leaked out of the blood capillaries and transports it to the pre-collector lymphatic

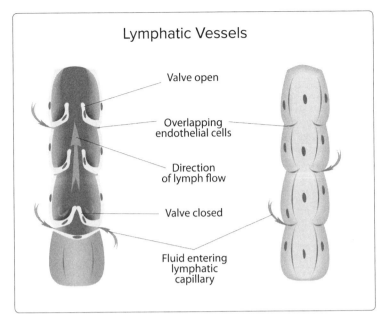

Lymphatic Vessels

Valve open

Overlapping endothelial cells

Direction of lymph flow

Valve closed

Fluid entering lymphatic capillary

Lymphatic vessels (longitudinal sections)

The lymph vessels are parallel to and travel with the veins, arteries and nerves throughout the entire body.

vessels, which are slightly larger in size. The pre-collectors then grow in size to become lymph collectors. These lymphatic vessels then carry the lymphatic fluid to the lymph nodes for filtering, and the fluid continues on to even larger lymphatic trunks. The lymphatic trunks return the fluid from your lower body and organs to your left subclavian vein. The fluid from your right arm, the right side of your chest, right shoulder and right side of your head returns to the heart via your right subclavian vein.

What is lymphedema?

Lymphedema is the abnormal accumulation of a protein-rich fluid called lymph. The proteins in the lymph are hydrophilic, which means they attract water and cause swelling.

Lymphedema presents as swelling, aching, heaviness, and pins and needles. It can occur in any area of your body, such as in the face, head, neck, genitals, breast or torso, but it is most common in the arms and legs. The look and feel of lymphedema can change over time. If it is left untreated, the extremity or the affected area can become enlarged, disfigured and painful. The condition can also cause a breakdown in the physical function of the area affected.

How does lymphedema develop?

When the lymphatic system is functioning well, the lymphatic vessels move excess fluid from areas of high concentration (the interstitial spaces) to areas of low concentration (the lymphatic vessels). However, when fluid is not moving well in the lymphatic system, it remains in the interstitial spaces rather than moving into the lymphatic

DID YOU KNOW?

The lymphatic system drains all of the lymph fluid from every area of your body, including the skin, muscles, joints and organs. It is analogous to a catch basin for your body.

capillaries. Eventually, an oversaturation in the interstitial spaces can occur, with proteins and leakage from the lymphatic vessels, resulting in lymphedema.

Comparing Blood Vessels and Lymphatic Vessels

BLOOD VESSELS	LYMPHATIC VESSELS
Pathway: heart ➡ arteries ➡ arterioles ➡ capillaries ➡ venules ➡ veins ➡ heart	Pathway: lymph capillaries* ➡ pre-collectors ➡ lymph collectors ➡ lymphatic trunks** ➡ lymph nodes ➡ lymphatic trunks ➡ subclavian veins
Blood follows a circular path	Lymphatic fluid flows in one direction, from interstitial spaces to subclavian veins, to re-enter the bloodstream
Carry nutrient- and oxygen-rich blood from the heart to the cells, then carry carbon dioxide and waste back to the lungs	Carry fluid and waste products from the tissue cells to the bloodstream
The exchange of oxygen and carbon dioxide occurs in the lungs; blood waste products are removed by the kidneys	Filtering and cleansing occurs during transport, when the lymph fluid passes through lymph nodes
Closed system	Open system
Pumped by the heart	No large pump — one-way valves are propelled by respiration, muscle contraction and the contraction of the larger lymph vessels
Carry fluid, red blood cells, plasma and blood gases (oxygen and carbon dioxide)	Carry fluid, white blood cells, protein, waste products and long-chain fatty acids
Functions: • Provide oxygen to cells • Return 80% to 90% of the blood back to the lungs • Facilitate gas exchange	Functions: • Capture the 10% to 20% of fluid that was not taken up by venous blood capillaries; remove proteins, bacteria, viruses and waste products from this fluid, then return it back to the blood • Transport immune cells (white blood cells) • Aid in the digestion and absorption of fats

* Single lymphatic vessels that begin in the gastrointestinal tract are called lacteals; vessels that begin in the interstitial spaces are lymph capillaries.
** The lymphatic trunks include the right lymphatic duct and the thoracic duct.

As you can see, the structure and function of blood vessels and lymphatic vessels are distinct, despite both being part of the circulatory system. It follows, then, that when something goes wrong with the functioning of these vessels, the treatments and nutritional supports must also be different. (See Part 3: Nutrition for Lymphedema for more information.)

What is the difference between edema and lymphedema?

Edema and lymphedema are two conditions that have many of the same characteristics but are often treated differently. Edema results when blood protein levels are too low and fluid moves from the blood into the tissues (or not enough fluid moves back to the blood). Lymphedema, on the other hand, is an accumulation of protein-rich lymphatic fluid in the body's interstitial spaces. For more information about these two conditions, see "Differences between Edema and Lymphedema," page 164. Consult your doctor or health-care specialist for more information and to determine the cause of your swelling.

What does the lymphatic system do?

The lymphatic system:

- Transports water and proteins; prevents swelling
- Acts as a vital component of your immune function
- Removes by-products of cell breakdown and debris from dead bacteria
- Flushes out toxins that do not belong in your body
- Transports long-chain fatty acids and fats from the gastrointestinal system back into the bloodstream

Sounding the Alarm

Lymph nodes are an important part of the immune system. As lymph enters a node, it is filtered. Infections (antigens) that have been carried into the node will be devoured by immune cells known as "big eaters" (macrophages). This will activate an alarm in other immune cells, such as B- and T-cells, that carry a memory of that specific infection. These cells then become activated to attack the infection. Some of them will circulate around the body to sound the alarm (a complete circuit will take between 12 and 24 hours) and others will rush to the site of the infection. When you have an infection, such as the flu, the lymph nodes in your neck may become swollen. This is, in part, due to the increase in the number of activated B- and T- cells in your lymph nodes. Once the infection is destroyed and the antigen depletes, the nodes return to normal size.

How might my lymphedema be different from other people's?

People with primary lymphedema can have swelling in any area of the body that has a lymphatic deficiency, such as one leg, both legs, one hand or the face, and it doesn't always have a symmetrical appearance. And some people who have primary lymphedema (see What Are the Different Types of Lymphedema?, page 22) experience poor lymphatic function throughout their entire body, sometimes called a "sluggish lymphatic system" — and this can cause swelling everywhere.

Others experience lymphedema in one area of the body. For example, after breast cancer, lymphedema may be seen in the arm, breast, upper back or side of the chest that is affected by the cancer. In individuals with cancer affecting the abdominal area or the reproductive organs, the swelling can be in both legs, the genitals and the lower abdominal area. In people with crush injuries, muscle tears or other injuries resulting in lymphatic damage, the swelling will be localized to the area that is injured and will likely extend down the limb. If the lymphedema is left untreated, it can also progress up the limb (toward the torso), depending on the extent of the damage to the lymphatic system and which pathways were damaged.

People with primary lymphedema can have swelling in any area of the body that has a lymphatic deficiency.

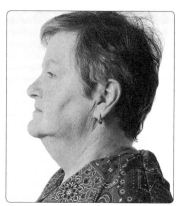

Head and neck lymphedema

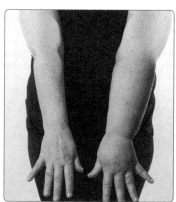

Arm lymphedema

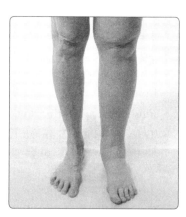

Leg lymphedema

What other vascular conditions could cause lymphedema to develop?

Vascular anomalies, such as vasodilation and angiogenesis (conditions that increase vascular flow to an area), can cause lymphedema if the lymphatic vessels in the area cannot keep up with the extra volume. Venous obstruction, such as a blood clot, can limit the ability of the veins to pump out the excess fluid that the arteries bring to a limb, for example, and this results in lymphedema because the lymphatics in the area are unable to compensate and clear the excess fluid. As you will read in Chapter 10, obesity can also be a cause of lymphedema.

What are the different types of lymphedema?

The two main types of lymphedema are known as primary and secondary lymphedema. Primary lymphedema is a lymphedema that develops because of a malformation of the lymphatic system in utero. This results in a deficiency of the lymphatic system, such as a reduced number of lymph nodes, a reduced number of lymphatic vessels or poorly organized lymphatic vessels. This form

DID YOU KNOW?

Primary lymphedema tends to appear in boys at birth and in girls and women during hormonal changes (puberty, pregnancy, menopause) — although there are exceptions. It can also present during times of physical and emotional stress, such as surgery or injury.

of lymphedema (with the resultant swelling) can be seen immediately at birth or at any time in a person's life. Primary lymphedema is a diagnosis of exclusion, meaning that all other major organ issues, such as heart, liver and kidney issues, have been ruled out before a definitive diagnosis of primary lymphedema can be made.

Secondary lymphedema occurs because of a physical or external injury to a healthy lymphatic system. This can be due to the removal of lymph nodes, cellulitis infection, the scarring of lymphatic vessels, surgical damage to lymphatic vessels, radiation damage to lymphatic vessels or nodes, crush injuries and many other reasons. When the lymphatic system is damaged, a blockage of fluid movement occurs. This is analogous to a car accident on a highway; when the accident on the highway blocks all the lanes, the highway begins to congest with vehicular traffic. The only way to get traffic moving again is to reroute it to an alternative road.

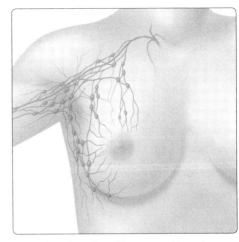
Lymph nodes of the arm and breast

How does radiation lead to lymphedema?

Radiation can cause an obstruction in the lymph vessels due to scarring and a thickening of the connective tissue in the vessel walls. It is also thought that radiation causes the skin cells to produce more collagen and that it removes the tufts in the skin where the blood vessels and lymphatics are.

In 1995, researchers from the United States showed that the blood vessels regress from the tufts, straighten out and dilate. We can hypothesize that this likely happens to the lymphatic vessels as well.

DID YOU KNOW?

One study by Vanderbilt University investigated the incidence rate of lymphedema in 81 patients with head and neck cancer: 75% (61 of 81 patients) had lymphedema. Of these 61 patients, 9.8% had external lymphedema, 39.4% had only internal lymphedema, and 50.8% had both internal and external lymphedema.

Impact of Radiation on Lymphedema Incidence Rates

RADIATION TARGET	LYMPHEDEMA INCIDENCE RATE
Breast/chest wall	14.5%
Breast/chest wall and supraclavicular (above the collarbone)	31.5%
Breast/chest wall and supraclavicular and posterior axillary boost (above the collarbone and including the underarm lymph nodes, or axilla)	41.4%
Genitourinary (genital and urinary systems)	16.0%
Gynecologic cancer	34.0%
Melanoma	50.0%

Source: *Shaitelman et al., 2015.*

What are the incidence rates of lymphedema in cancer patients?

The following table illustrates incidence rates of lymphedema in common cancer conditions:

TYPE OF CANCER	TYPE OF TREATMENT	LYMPHEDEMA INCIDENCE RATE
Endometrial cancer	Any	1.0%
Head and neck cancer	Any	4.0%
Prostate cancer	Any	4.0%
Melanoma	Sentinel lymph node dissection (SLND) Lymph node dissection (LND)	4.1% 9.0%
Breast cancer	Sentinel lymph node dissection (SLND) Axillary lymph node dissection (ALND)	6.3% 22.3%
Bladder cancer	Any	16.0%
Penile cancer	Any	21.0%
Gynecological cancer	Any	25.0%
Cervical cancer	Any	27.0%
Vulvar cancer	Any	30.0%
Sarcoma cancer	Any	30.0%

Source: *Shaitelman et al., 2015.*

What are the stages of lymphedema?

- **Stage 0:** This is the difficult-to-see (subclinical) stage and the earliest presentation of lymphedema. There is no measurable swelling. Symptoms often reported include heaviness, aching, and pins and needles. You can be in this stage for months or years before swelling develops.

- **Stage 1:** Your swelling is detectable and measurable. The swelling subsides with the elevation of your affected limb. The swelling tends to come and go. There may also be pitting edema at this stage.

- **Early stage 2:** Elevating your limb is ineffective and rarely helps to reduce swelling. Pitting edema will more typically occur at this stage.

- **Late stage 2:** Tissue fibrosis is more evident in this period. Pitting edema may or may not occur.

- **Stage 3:** Skin changes, such as thickening, darker skin (hyperpigmentation), skin folds, fat deposits and warty overgrowths, start to develop. Small pores in the skin can develop, and clear lymphatic fluid can leak out. The limb is hard and fibrotic, and there is no pitting at this stage.

How does lymphedema progress?

Overall, as lymphedema progresses, you will see a steady increase in swelling and, potentially, pain. The progression of lymphedema can lead to thickened skin, a change in tissue density, reduced joint function, reduced ability to complete the activities of daily living, altered walking and dexterity, and reduced balance.

What are the other aspects of health that are affected by lymphedema?

People who have lymphedema can be impacted by other health-related complications, such as:

- Reduced activity level
- Reduced general health
- Cellulitis
- Obesity
- Cardiovascular disease and hypertension
- Psychological impact

What are the different ways lymphedema can be measured?

Lymphedema can be measured in a number of different ways.

- **Circumference measurement:** This technique uses a measuring tape to measure the circumference (girth) of your limb at multiple points. In many cases, if the limb's girth is larger than the unaffected limb by $3/4$ inch (2 cm) in three or more consecutive spots, a diagnosis of lymphedema will be given.

- **Water displacement:** This technique uses a large cylinder filled with water. You place your arm or leg with lymphedema into the cylinder, and the amount of water displaced by the limb is measured. This value is the volume of limb swelling.

- **Perimetry:** This is a noninvasive device called a perimeter that uses infrared light to measure the perimeter of the limb; this number is used to calculate the volume of the limb.

- **Bioelectric impedance analysis:** This technique measures the flow of an electrical current through the body and is used to determine the amount of fluid in a region of the body.

How can I use self-measurement to tell if I'm having a flare-up?

Learning how to measure your own lymphedema limb can be very helpful in determining if you are having a flare-up. You and your lymphedema therapist may use the term "flare-up" to describe any increase in your lymphedema after a period of stability (see "Who is qualified to help me manage my lymphedema?" on page 28).

DID YOU KNOW?

The causes of lymphedema are estimated to be:

- Obesity: 50%
- Cancer: 15%
- Disability: 8%
- Surgery: 4%
- Primary: 2%

Overall, as lymphedema progresses, you will see a steady increase in swelling and, potentially, pain.

DID YOU KNOW?

You can monitor the size of your limb at home with the use of a measuring tape. See page 26 for a guide to measurement.

Typically, you can learn to measure your own limb with a little bit of practice. Your lymphedema therapist can tell you how often to measure, but if you're stable, measuring about once a month is fine. It's important to measure the same locations each time. The pictures that follow are suggested locations; however, if you have a scar or mole, you can use these as your landmarks for measuring. Take four or five measurements of your limb. Use the same spots each day (see image below), keeping these key considerations in mind:

- Use the same measurement locations.
- Measure once a month if your lymphedema is stable.
- Measure at the same time each day that you measure.
- Measure a bare limb (do not measure over bandaging or other compression).
- Avoid pulling the measuring tape too tightly around your limb; it should sit flat on the surface of your skin (it should not "pucker" the skin).
- Measure more frequently if you are introducing a new exercise or activity, returning to work, making changes to your diet or changing the type of compression garments you're wearing.

The overall goal is to maintain a stable limb that does not increase in size. Monitoring your size can help you determine how your lymphedema responds to various situations and treatments.

Self Measurements

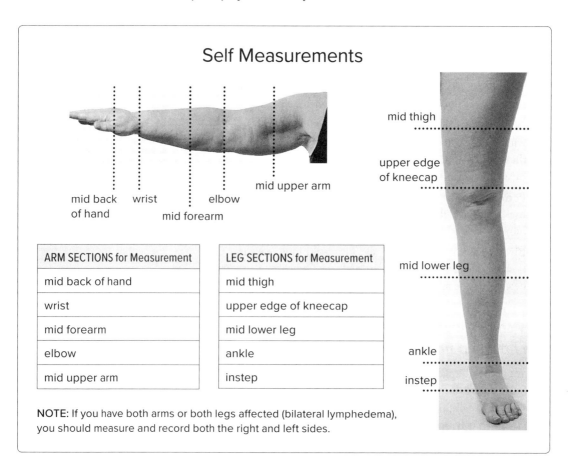

ARM SECTIONS for Measurement	LEG SECTIONS for Measurement
mid back of hand	mid thigh
wrist	upper edge of kneecap
mid forearm	mid lower leg
elbow	ankle
mid upper arm	instep

NOTE: If you have both arms or both legs affected (bilateral lymphedema), you should measure and record both the right and left sides.

What are the different types of tests used to determine where the abnormality exists in the lymphatic system?

There are a number of different tools that can be used, including:

- **Lymphoscintigraphy:** A radioactive tracer is injected into the skin between the toes or fingers and imaging is used to visualize the tracer as it travels through the lymphatics. A slow uptake of the tracer or no movement of the tracer would indicate lymphatic deficiency.
- **Near-infrared fluorescence imaging:** This technique can be used to diagnose early lymphedema. Indocyanine green (ICG) dye is injected under the skin and the uptake of the ICG by the lymphatics can be visualized with dim near-infrared light. Lymphatic function and dysfunction can be determined using this technique.
- **Magnetic resonance imaging (MRI):** Magnetic-resonance-based lymphangiography can be used to visualize the lymphatic system. A gadolinium-based contrast agent is injected into the skin and its tracking through the system is visualized using MRI.

My family member has primary lymphedema. Does this mean I might get it, too?

It is estimated that approximately 5% to 10% of primary lymphedema cases are hereditary. The incidence is higher in females than males, with females presenting mostly at puberty and males presenting mostly at birth. There are seven known genes implicated in the incidence of primary lymphedema. The research in this area began only in the early 2000s, but research continues to look at the genetic link to lymphedema.

Are there genetic links to cancer-related secondary lymphedema?

Studies have identified genes that are known to impact lymphatic development, and the results of these studies may explain why only some patients develop cancer-related lymphedema after treatments for their cancer. In a study of 59 women with breast-cancer-related secondary lymphedema, several gene mutations were found. Some of these genes are involved in regulating the body's inflammatory response. Read more about inflammation and lymphedema in Chapter 12.

When should I get treatment for my lymphedema?

For the treatment of lymphedema to be most effective, it should be done as early as possible. Early treatment helps prevent chronic changes, such as fibrosis of the tissue or fat deposition in the swollen limb, and it can slow the progression to more advanced stages of the disease.

LIVING WITH LYMPHEDEMA

"You have to figure out what works for you and put it all together. Everyone has a different experience."

DID YOU KNOW?

Lymph nodes do not regenerate, but lymphatic vessels might. Lymphangiogenesis — the creation of new lymphatic vessels — has been seen in animal models.

DID YOU KNOW?

Liao's study showed that at 1 year, 21% had more severe lymphedema, and at 3 years, 34% had more severe lymphedema; thus, treating mild lymphedema is imperative to reducing the severity of the disease.

Are there medications or pills that I can take to treat my lymphedema?

No specific medications exist today to treat lymphedema. However, people with lymphedema are often given a trial of diuretic medication. Diuretics simply remove water from the blood to reduce blood volume. Initially, diuretics may be effective, but the benefits are typically not sustained over time. Diuretics can also cause electrolyte imbalances because they remove potassium from the body. Diuretics are thought to concentrate the proteins in the lymph, which can stimulate fibrosis of the tissues and potentially make you more susceptible to cellulitis infections. Specialists recommend avoiding long-term diuretic use for lymphedema.

What is the treatment for lymphedema?

The benefits of early diagnosis and intervention in lymphedema have been heavily researched, and it is known that early intervention can often minimize the progression of the condition. The treatment is divided into two phases: the initial intensive phase and the maintenance phase. The gold standard of care is complete decongestive therapy, also known as CDT, which consists of these four key elements:

1. Skin care
2. Manual lymphatic drainage
3. Compression therapy
   a. Bandaging (intensive phase)
   b. Compression garments (maintenance phase)
4. Exercise

The goal of CDT is to reduce your limb volume in as short a time as possible and then to maintain it. In 2013, researchers Liao and colleagues determined that the baseline limb volume prior to CDT was correlated to the length of time a patient had lymphedema. If patients are diagnosed earlier, lymphedema management can start before the size of the limb increases. The longer the lymphedema persists, the more severe the lymphedema becomes.

Many research studies have shown that CDT reduces the symptoms of lymphedema and improves quality of life.

Who is qualified to help me manage my lymphedema?

Lymphedema therapists have a special certification called complete decongestive therapy (CDT) certification. In Canada and the United States, it is a postgraduate certification that can be done by a physiotherapist (also called a physical therapist) or assistant (PT assistant), occupational therapist (OT) or assistant (OT assistant), massage therapist (RMT), nurse (RN), athletic therapist (ATC) or doctor (MD). Practitioners must have a minimum of 135 hours of CDT training with at least 90 hours of practical hands-on training in class before they can be certified.

Accepted Credentials

Professional titles may vary. These are the three most common credentials to look for:

- **CDT:** complete decongestive therapist, combined lymphedema therapist or comprehensive lymphedema therapist (CDT is also the name of the therapy called complete decongestive therapy)
- **CLT:** certified lymphedema therapist
- **DLT:** decongestive lymphedema therapist

CDT is the most commonly used credential, but most CDTs, CLTs and DLTs refer to themselves simply as "lymphedema therapists." In this book, a "lymphedema therapist" refers to a therapist certified in complete decongestive therapy.

Lymphedema therapists have the necessary training, education and skill required to manage disorders of the lymphatic system effectively.

At this time, there is no regulation of lymphedema therapists, so some health-care workers will accept lymphedema patients even though they do not hold the proper certification to treat them effectively. It is the recommendation of the National Lymphedema Network (NLN) that you seek the care of a therapist certified in CDT. Lymphedema therapists have the necessary training, education and skill required to manage disorders of the lymphatic system effectively.

A therapist who has completed the proper training will use the acronym CDT, CLT or DLT after their name and their professional title — for example, a physiotherapist who has completed the certification will have "PT, CDT" after their name. Check the credentials of your prospective health professional to make sure you get the right help for your lymphedema.

To find a lymphedema therapist in the United States, visit the NLN website or call the organization to access the names of local therapists who are registered with them. In Canada, contact your provincial lymphedema association. Alternatively, you can call or visit the websites of training schools for lymphedema; the major schools will each have a list of therapists who have trained with them.

What can I do to help manage my lymphedema?

Self-management needs to be a part of all lymphedema treatments. It is important that you take control of the condition and work together with your lymphedema therapist to achieve the best outcome. Always work with a lymphedema therapist during the intensive (or first) phase of treatment, when the goal is reduction. Use these sessions to learn about your lymphedema, the lymphatic system, and which pathways work best for your individual needs.

DID YOU KNOW?

It is important that you be an informed and involved member of your health-care team. You should always understand what treatments will be done and how your goals will be met. Your health-care team should give you lots of information about your condition and how it affects your overall health, including other parts of your body (such as joints and organs). You should also understand how each treatment might impact your illness and symptoms.

Make sure you understand the importance of self-management and the possible outcomes if you stop self-treating. Your complete program for self-management should include all the components of CDT outlined in this book. Other components of physical therapy may also need to be added to your personalized program to help you achieve optimal results.

Part 2 of this book goes into more detail about the various self-care strategies that may improve your symptoms and slow the progression of the disease.

Training Schools for Lymphedema Therapists

Integrated Lymph Drainage: www.torontolymphocare.com

Academy of Lymphatic Studies: www.acols.com

Casley-Smith International: www.casleysmithinternational.org

International Lymphedema and Wound Training Institute: www.ilwti.com

Klose Training & Consulting: www.klosetraining.com

LymphEd: www.lymphed.com

National Lymphedema Network: www.lymphnet.org

Norton School of Lymphatic Therapy: www.nortonschool.com

Dr. Vodder School International: www.vodderschool.com

CHAPTER 2

Lymphedema Risk Reduction

Can lymphedema be prevented? This is a critical question that every person who has ever been told they are at risk for lymphedema has probably asked their health-care professional. At this time, there is insufficient evidence to show that lymphedema can be prevented. A number of the strategies outlined in this chapter have been developed by lymphedema therapists in clinical practice over many decades. These are guidelines to help you reduce your risk of developing lymphedema.

Many of the guidelines outlined below are derived from common sense and are based on the physiological functions of the body, the circulatory system and the lymphatic system. The goal is to reduce the stress on the lymphatics and prevent lymphedema from developing. More research is being conducted to prove or disprove these strategies; until then, they represent the current best practices for lymphedema risk reduction. It is important to keep in mind that your situation is unique and will require unique risk-reduction measures based on your lifestyle.

DID YOU KNOW?

People who are at risk of developing lymphedema are those who have had lymph nodes removed or radiated, people whose lymphatic systems have been damaged, those with past cellulitis infections and those with conditions that promote limb swelling.

Not every person who has lymph nodes removed develops lymphedema. Several studies have tried to determine if there is a way to predict who is at risk.

Strategies to Reduce Your Risk of Developing Lymphedema

Minimize Lymph Node Removal

There are several cancer types that can spread to lymph nodes. In broad terms, they are the carcinomas (cancers from epithelial cells). These cancers include adenocarcinoma (a type of cancer that starts in the mucous glands inside of organs), prostate, bladder, lymph, breast, ovary, cervix, and head and neck. Removing the lymph nodes is done to reduce the risk of cancer spreading (metastasizing).

Not every person who has lymph nodes removed develops lymphedema. Several studies have tried to determine if there is a way to predict who is at risk for developing lymphedema, what the risk factors are, and what can be done to reduce the risk. Many of these studies are done in breast cancer patients who are at risk of developing arm lymphedema after lymph nodes are removed from the armpit (axilla).

One risk factor that presents itself repeatedly in the cancer and lymphedema research is the removal of a higher number of lymph nodes. Researchers from Vanderbilt University and the University of Missouri recruited 138 women for a study. The data they collected showed that the patients who had axillary lymph node dissection versus sentinel lymph node dissection (see below) were more likely to develop lymphedema. It's important to note that the primary decision regarding how many lymph nodes to remove should be based on the best treatment for your cancer — and not on preventing lymphedema. This is at the discretion of your surgeon during your operation.

The number of lymph nodes removed might be considered an unmodifiable risk factor, since it's largely up to your surgeon during the surgery — but this shouldn't prevent you from having a conversation about lymphedema risk with your surgeon before the operation. The following list of risk factors can be considered modifiable because they are more within your control.

Sentinel Node Testing

There are many different techniques used in cancer treatment. Some surgical options, such as the use of sentinel node testing, may have an impact on lymphedema. This surgical technique involves the injection of a dye at the site of the cancer tumor. The first node or nodes that pick up the dye (the sentinel nodes) are typically the lymph nodes removed, but this depends on the type of cancer and other factors. If the cancer is in multiple nodes, such as in the armpit (axilla), more extensive node removal may be needed, but this, too, is dependent on other factors.

In a study in 2013, Bernas and colleagues found that removing only the sentinel node lowers the risk of lymphedema. However, it is not always possible to remove only the sentinel node, and more extensive node removal is highly dependent on the stage of cancer. Early cancer detection leads to less extensive node removal and thus lowers the risk of lymphedema.

Educate Yourself Early

Education regarding key risk-reduction practices and treatment options is important, especially for patients in any phase of cancer treatment. In 2002, Box and colleagues showed that if education about lymphedema and its risk-reduction practices occurred early, patients had a decreased incidence of lymphedema. These researchers saw a lymphedema incidence rate of 11% in the education group, while the control group (which received no education) saw a 30% rate of lymphedema.

Intervene Early

As with any type of medical treatment, early detection and intervention can lead to more manageable symptoms and potentially prevent a full lymphedema diagnosis. In 2008, Stout Gergich and colleagues showed that there are some benefits to early intervention in lymphedema. The researchers used compression sleeves on patients as soon as there was detectable swelling — instead of waiting until a 10% volume increase was detected (a practice outlined in many clinical guidelines). When the compression sleeves were used for a period of 4 weeks and then removed, patients were able to maintain the reduction in size for 5 months following this treatment.

Take Precautions Before and During Air Travel

Many people consider air travel a trigger for lymphedema, as there are many reports of at-risk individuals developing lymphedema after flying in planes. Air travel involves low oxygen levels, low cabin pressure, decreased activity and dehydration; these risks may be enough to trigger lymphedema. In 1996, Casley-Smith showed a relationship between air travel and the onset of lymphedema, with 6% of people who responded to a questionnaire stating that they developed lymphedema due to flying. In 2005, Hayes and colleagues found an incidence rate two to five times higher in people following air travel. More research is required to determine if there is a conclusive link between air travel and lymphedema. However, based on physiological principles, it is possible, and steps should be taken to minimize the risk.

> ## LIVING WITH LYMPHEDEMA
> *"I've talked to a pilot; it's not so much the altitude changes — it's how the pilot goes down. Rapid altitude changes are too fast for your impaired lymphatic system."*

FAQ

Q. How can I protect myself while flying, to prevent lymphedema?

A. If you are at risk of lymphedema, you should take precautions before you fly (such as proper hydration and self-MLD; see "Self-MLD," page 52) and during flying (such as moving and exercising limbs and using bandages or compression sleeves; see chapters 5 and 6). It is imperative that lymphedema sleeves fit properly, as poorly fitting sleeves can trigger the development of lymphedema.

Unless specified by your medical team, there is no reason to restrict air travel following breast cancer surgery or any other surgery where nodes are removed. And although there's no guarantee that you won't develop lymphedema after flying, if you bandage or use compression garments, you can help reduce the risk.

Limit Needle Punctures or Blood Draws

Any damage to the skin or the skin barrier can increase the risk of infection. As a result, precautions should be taken to try to avoid any type of needle puncture or blood draw. The risk of infection is higher in those who have previously had skin punctures. Puncturing the skin is also thought to increase the risk of inflammation in the at-risk limb, which could trigger lymphedema or worsen it.

Individuals at risk for arm lymphedema should avoid any type of needle puncture or blood draw if at all possible. For those with the risk of lymphedema in both arms, veins or arteries in the foot can be used for blood draws or infusions.

Limit the Use of Blood Pressure Cuffs

Similarly to needle punctures and blood draws, the use of blood pressure cuffs can increase the incidence of inflammation of a limb that is at risk of developing lymphedema. Use of a blood pressure cuff is necessary for many patients who monitor their blood pressure or heart health, but care is required to determine which limb is best to use. The high pressure applied by the cuff is thought to temporarily collapse the lymphatic vessels and promote local inflammation. It has been speculated that increased venous pressure may increase lymph production and cause swelling. This is another area that requires further research, as there are very few quality studies in this area.

Limit Repetitive Limb Movements

Repetitive movements increase blood flow to the contracting muscles in order to fuel the repeated activity. This, in turn, causes the collection of more lymph in the limb, which can aggravate the existing lymphedema or initiate the development of lymphedema. Repeated motions — such as those used in everyday job duties or household duties — could be triggers for increased swelling. Examples of repeated motions could include repetitive lifting, chopping, hammering, etc. It is important to break up repetitive activities into small, manageable chunks. Repetitive activities should be spread out over the course of the day or over several days if possible.

Avoid Temperature Extremes

It is important to avoid sudden or prolonged temperature changes that are either hot or cold. It's best to avoid the following examples of exposures that can increase lymph formation:

- Sunburns
- Exposure to extreme cold
- The submerging of an at-risk limb in water warmer than 102°F (38.9°C)
- Hot packs and heating pads (which cause the blood vessels to release more fluid into the interstitial spaces)
- Cold packs (which, when removed from the limb, cause blood to be pumped quickly to the area to warm it up; this, in turn, results in excess lymph in the interstitial spaces)

An understanding of how the lymphatic and circulatory systems work guides our recommendations in this area.

Protect from and Treat Injuries and Infections

Whenever possible, it is important to avoid activities that could increase the chances of injury to the skin of an affected limb. You should protect your skin from injury and keep cuts clean and covered to prevent infection. In 2016, Asdourian and colleagues found that a history of previous infections was the most clearly established risk factor for developing lymphedema.

An increased number of bouts of severe cellulitis will damage the lymphatic system further, worsen arm or leg lymphedema, and increase the risk of infections (see Chapter 3 for more information about cellulitis and other skin issues). Cellulitis can occur in any part of the body affected by lymphedema. If any signs or symptoms of cellulitis occur, seek immediate medical attention. Bacteria can spread quickly and can enter the bloodstream, leading to major complications that can worsen lymphedema and that might even be life-threatening.

Achieve and Maintain an Ideal Body Weight

Having a high body weight and body mass index (BMI) is another risk factor for lymphedema. Increased body fat limits the ability of lymphatic fluid to move, and this results in higher amounts of fluid in the tissue. The lymphatic vessels are thought to be distorted by the deposits of fat cells around the layers of skin. In general, a greater concentration of fat cells impedes the movement of lymphatic fluid and causes swelling to occur. It is important to maintain a healthy body weight and BMI to reduce the possibility of developing lymphedema. (See Appendix 2: BMI Table, page 244, for more information.)

> ➡ **PRO TIP**
>
> You may not have control over how many lymph nodes are removed in your surgery, but you do have some control over your body weight. Even if you have a large number of nodes removed, you may still be able to reduce your modifiable risk factors, such as being overweight.

Body Weight and Cancer Treatment

In the study from Vanderbilt University and the University of Missouri that examined the types of lymph node removal, researchers discovered that — no matter what type of lymph node dissection was done, either axillary or sentinel — a BMI of 30 or greater was still a significant risk factor for the development of lymphedema.

While there may not be much time to lose weight before a cancer surgery (and certainly there's no time before an unexpected infection or injury), it would be prudent to see a dietitian prior to a planned surgery. A dietitian can start you on healthy weight-loss strategies preoperatively, which could reduce the risk of lymphedema caused by surgery. A dietitian can also continue to monitor your weight and diet post-surgery. Make sure to track your weight and monitor your limb for swelling for the first 18 months post-surgery.

Obesity Itself as a Risk Factor

When it comes to predicting which patients undergoing cancer treatment might develop lymphedema, body weight consistently appears as a risk factor. We can make a prediction that body weight could also influence the development of lymphedema in other scenarios as well, such as infections and injury to the lymphatic system, although this has not been scientifically researched as of yet.

In a 2012 letter to the editor of the *New England Journal of Medicine*, Greene and associates describe that obesity — not cancer or lymph node injury or removal — is associated with lower-limb lymphedema. In their study, the researchers examined the legs of 15 obese people (12 women and three men). Five were found to have lymphedema and 10 did not. They determined that the greater the obesity, the greater the likelihood that lymphedema would develop. The five people who had lymphedema had a BMI range of 59.7 to 88.1, whereas the 10 people who didn't have lymphedema had a BMI range of 30.7 to 53.3. In this examination, extreme obesity (also called Class 3 obesity) appeared to be the primary link to the occurrence of lymphedema. The theory behind this connection is that:

1. Compression or inflammation by fat tissue may impair the functioning of the lymphatic system.

2. There is an increase in the production of lymphatic fluid because of the larger limb and the excess fatty tissue.

The good news is that these researchers speculate that weight loss has the potential to reverse the lymphedema.

A Give-and-Take Relationship

In a Special Topic article from 2014, Mehrara and colleagues describe the relationship between lymphedema and obesity as a "reciprocal" relationship. In this vicious cycle, obesity leads to lymphedema, which leads to obesity, which leads to more lymphedema. The relationship looks like this:

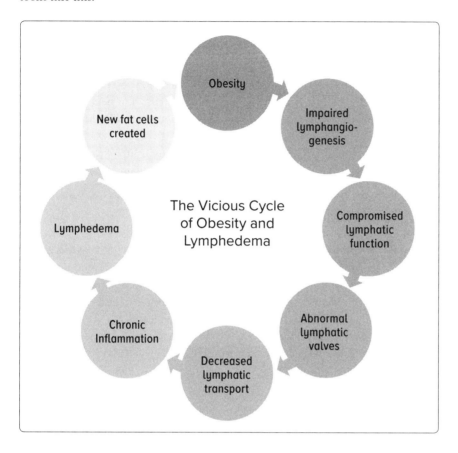

Preliminary studies have shown that some of these changes can be reversible with calorie restriction and weight loss.

Decision-Making about Risk Factors

It's important to remember that some risk factors are within your control and some are not. In a 2015 study looking at risk factors for developing lymphedema in cancer patients, researchers in Romania discussed how to reduce risk. Factors that they concluded can reduce the risk of lymphedema include:

- Opting for sentinel node resection versus axillary node resection when possible
- Avoiding post-treatment biopsy when possible

It's important to remember that some risk factors are within your control and some are not.

- Limiting total dose of radiation treatment to 45 to 50 Gy
- Limiting radiation on overweight patients and patients over 55 years of age
- Starting physical exercise a short time after surgery
- Self-massaging (known as manual lymphatic drainage)
- Compressive bandaging
- Ensuring good daily hygiene
- Consuming a healthy diet

It's important to remember that the main aim of cancer treatment is to cure the cancer, not to prevent lymphedema.

The first four items on this list should be discussed with your cancer care team; you will need to consider your overall cancer treatment and not just your lymphedema risk. The next four factors are addressed in detail in Part 2 of this book, and a healthy diet for lymphedema is discussed in Part 3.

It's important to remember that the main aim of cancer treatment is to cure the cancer, not to prevent lymphedema.

The Bottom Line

Research continues to take place on which risk factors may trigger lymphedema development. Education is the key to prevention in many medical conditions, and it is no different for lymphedema. The guidelines summarized here should be taken into consideration by any individual at risk for developing lymphedema.

- Educate yourself about lymphedema.
- If you see swelling, don't delay; get help as soon as you can.
- Take precautions before and during air travel.
- Limit needle punctures and blood draws in at-risk limbs.
- Be cautious with blood pressure cuffs on at-risk limbs.
- Avoid repetitive limb movements.
- Avoid extreme temperatures, including hot and cold packs.
- Protect your skin from injury and infections and treat appropriately when they occur.
- Achieve and maintain an ideal body weight.

PART 2
Self-Care for Lymphedema

CHAPTER 3

Skin Care

The skin is the largest organ of the body. It plays a vital role in general health, it protects us from infection, and it creates a barrier between our internal organs/tissues and our environment. Proper skin care is important for everyone, but it is critically important for people living with lymphedema, as injury to the skin can lead to painful and debilitating cellulitis infections.

LIVING WITH LYMPHEDEMA

"I got stung by a bee on my finger on my lymphedema hand; it got really swollen and red. Thankfully, I always carry Benadryl or Reactine and I think that helped. I was told to make a line on my finger and if the redness traveled up my hand and crossed the line, I should go to the hospital."

Why Skin Care Is Important

- The skin contains 70% of the lymphatic vessels, so having healthy, supple skin is essential for the movement of lymphatic fluid. Compromised skin reduces the lymphatic system's ability to clear excess fluid from an area.

- If you have an injury such as a scratch, bug bite or sunburn, your body transports immune cells to that area through the lymphatic and circulatory systems. These immune cells, along with blood and lymphatic fluid, reach the area and increase the lymphatic volume — but in lymphedema, excess lymph cannot leave the area and swelling begins. Protecting your skin from injury is your first line of defense.

- The skin is also a barrier against the outside world. When it is dry and cracked, bacteria can enter through the skin and cause infection. In a lymphedema limb, your immune response is impaired and you are more prone to infection, which can lead to painful and debilitating cellulitis.

Soft, supple skin allows the body to clear out excess lymphatic fluid.

Intact skin that is free of cuts and cracks provides a natural barrier to bacteria and protection against infection.

Preventing bug bites, burns and cuts keeps limbs from being overrun with white blood cells and lymphatic fluid.

The Triple Goals of
Skin Care in Lymphedema

The Acid Mantle

In a research article published in 2013, investigators from the United States examined the science of the skin. Interestingly, the skin is actually acidic in its pH level; this is called the acid mantle. In order to keep our skin healthy, we should try to maintain that acidic nature. In many diseases affecting the skin, such as dermatitis, the pH of the skin is often altered, which leads to dryness and cracking and leaves the skin susceptible to infection.

The normal pH of the skin is between 4 and 6, and the internal environment of your body ranges from 7 to 9. To keep your skin healthy, you should aim to maintain the normal skin pH of 4 to 6. If skin pH becomes more neutral, or alkaline, dry, flaking skin can develop. Skin pH also controls the amount and type of bacteria on the skin's surface. Some bacteria thrive in the acidic environment, such as some types of streptococcus bacteria. When an environment becomes closer to neutral pH, bacteria such as *Staphylococcus aureus* can live on the skin. These bacteria have the potential to damage your health; if they enter your body through a compromised skin barrier, they multiply and can damage internal tissues such as your organs.

It has been speculated that people with lymphedema have skin that falls outside the normal pH range, moving toward the alkaline level and causing dry skin. Maintaining the skin pH has been credited with maintaining the skin barrier, the health of skin cells, and bacterial defense.

Finding Low-pH Skin Care Products

The goal when choosing skin care products is to pick products that maintain the acidic nature of the skin. Very few soaps, cleansers and moisturizers are available in the United States and Canada that have a low pH. There are no standards for manufacturers to ensure that skin care products are within the acidic pH range. Also, it's important to note that products with the same name may contain different ingredients in different countries (these are based on government regulations); therefore, the pH levels of a single product may be different in different countries.

Industry and government regulations don't require that pH levels are listed on skin care products, so how do you know what to buy? It is helpful to call the manufacturer of the products you are using to find out the pH level, although not all major skin care manufacturers provide this information through their customer service representatives. Outside of calling the manufacturer, you can spot-test new products on a small area of your healthy skin for several days to determine your individual response to these products. This won't tell you the pH of the product, but it will determine if you react to it or not.

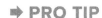
Cleansers can be divided into soap-based and non-soap-based cleaners (the latter of these are called syndets). Syndets are synthetic detergent–based bars or liquids and are acidic (having a pH less than 7). Soap-based cleansers are usually more alkaline (with a pH of about 10). As a result, soap-based products tend to be more irritating and drying to the skin than syndets. It is very important to use skin care products that are close to your skin's natural pH and that work for your individual skin type, as healthy skin pH levels can help maintain healthy and supple skin and prevent infection. The tables in Appendix 1: pH Levels of Skin Care Products (page 241) list the pH levels of commonly found skin care products available in the United States and Canada. The acid mantle tested at pH 4.71 ± 0.01.

Choosing Skin Care Products

When it comes to skin care, we need to examine the types of products used on the skin. It is important to read labels and pay attention to the acid and alkaline levels of soaps and lotions. Here are some tips to help you find the right skin care products:

- Choose petroleum-free products. Petroleum can break down the fibers of your compression garments.
- Choose unscented lotion with a slightly acidic pH level.
- Do not choose your products based on price. Price is not a good indicator of pH quality. Some expensive products on the market are poor choices from a pH standpoint.

Treatment of Other Skin Issues

It is also important to consider the individual ingredients in your skin care products. The table on page 43 lists a few examples of skin conditions and some ingredients that may be helpful in the treatment of those conditions. If you have a skin condition, bring it to the attention of your physician, and you may even need to speak to a skin specialist (a dermatologist). Make sure to treat skin issues quickly and effectively so that the skin can return to its naturally acidic pH level and so that normal functions can be restored.

Research Review: Skin Infections

There is significant research to show that people who have recurrent infections may benefit from long-term preventive antibiotic use to avoid infection. A study in India from 2004 randomly assigned 150 lymphedema patients with recurrent skin infections to one of

Skin Issues and Skin Care Product Ingredients for Treatment

SKIN ISSUE	INGREDIENT FOR TREATMENT
Dry skin. Ingredient at right helps return the skin pH to its acidic level	Lactic acid
Hyperkeratotic skin desquamation. Ingredients at right help remove dry/thick discolored skin that can be a result of long-standing chronic lymphedema.	Lactic acid Urea (also called carbamide) Ceramides Glycerin Dimethicone (also called polydimethyl- siloxane and dimethylpolysiloxane) Olive fruit oil Salicylic acid
Dermatitis. Ingredient at right reduces inflammation.	Topical steroids

Sources: *Rawlings et al., 1996; Fife et al., 2017.*

five groups. They all learned to perform self-management of their lymphedema limbs, which included nail care, proper washing of the skin, drying between the creases and toes, and the use of salicylic-acid ointments (6%) on the skin. The second part of the study assigned participants to one of five additional treatments: taking oral penicillin, taking oral diethylcarbamazine, taking both penicillin and diethylcarbamazine, applying framycetin ointment or applying a placebo ointment. The greatest reduction in infection rates was seen in the group that was given oral penicillin. However, when the medication was discontinued after 1 year, the cycles of infection returned. This research suggests that preventive oral antibiotics may be needed for more than 1 year in those with recurrent skin infections.

Preventive oral antibiotics may be needed for more than 1 year in those with recurrent skin infections.

But long-term use of antibiotics is not the only way to prevent infection. Other research cited in the study above has shown that those who did intensive self-management had fewer infections compared to the previous year, which suggests that self-care can also lessen the burden of infection in lymphedema.

Dealing with Recurring Skin Infections

If you have experienced at least three skin infections in 1 year, speak with your doctor about whether oral antibiotics should be used as a preventive strategy. Consider using the self-management strategies of exercise, skin care (see "Skin Care Strategies," page 46), manual lymphatic drainage and compression therapy to help prevent infections; reducing the swelling will lower the risk of infection and create a healthier internal environment.

Infections leave behind hidden damage. Each cycle of infection creates scar tissue, which damages more lymphatic vessels and impairs your lymphatic system. This impairment, in turn, usually leads to a worsening of the lymphedema. One cycle of infection is known to predispose you to future cycles of infection, so practice prevention!

Consider using the self-management strategies of exercise, skin care, manual lymphatic drainage and compression therapy to help prevent infections.

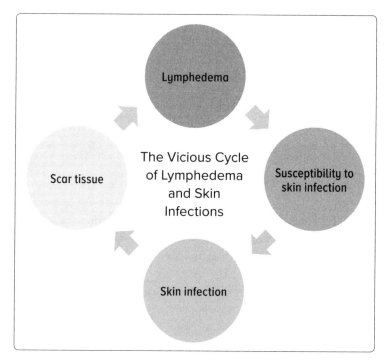

The Vicious Cycle of Lymphedema and Skin Infections

Lymphedema → Susceptibility to skin infection → Skin infection → Scar tissue → Lymphedema

Cellulitis

Cellulitis occurs when bacteria have entered through the skin and cause acute inflammation of the skin and underlying tissues; the bacteria are commonly a *Streptococcus* or *Staphylococcus* bacteria strain. The lower leg is the most affected site and is responsible for 75% to 90% of all cases of cellulitis. Lymphedema has been shown to be one of the biggest risk factors for developing cellulitis.

Damage to the skin can be the result of animal scratches or bites, cuts in the skin, dry skin, nail biting, cut cuticles or abrasions to the skin. The cellulitis can grow in size and become a large wound.

From person to person, the signs and symptoms can vary; likewise, one person's cellulitis signs and symptoms may vary from one infection to the next. Symptoms can develop over days or in a very short period of time (such as less than an hour). The symptoms of cellulitis can include all or just a few of the ones listed here:

- Pain
- Redness
- Warmth
- Swelling
- Blisters
- Rash
- Lines of redness (streaking)

When bacteria have entered the bloodstream, symptoms progress to more flu-like symptoms, such as chills, fever, headache and vomiting.

Cellulitis can be a life-threatening condition, and immediate medical attention is needed. Go to your doctor or local emergency room as soon as symptoms of infection are noticed. Depending on the severity of your symptoms, intravenous (IV) or oral antibiotics may be administered. Oral antibiotics are slower to enter the bloodstream and it takes several doses before they are able to kill the bacteria. Intravenous antibiotics are administered into the bloodstream and start working much more quickly.

Cellulitis in Arm Lymphedema

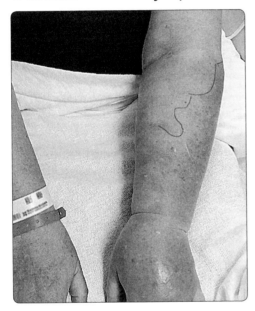

A pen is used by hospital staff to mark the leading edge of the infection. If the red area spreads past the pen marks, the infection is continuing to spread.

Skin Changes with Lymphedema

The skin changes that happen with lymphedema are more common in people who have had undiagnosed or untreated lymphedema for years. Individuals who treat their lymphedema early and continue to do self-management are less likely to have one of the many potential chronic skin changes seen in long-standing untreated lymphedema. These changes include:

- Leakage of lymphatic fluid from pores in the skin (lymphorrhea)
- Skin breakdown wounds
- Mole or wart overgrowths
- Dense, thickened areas of skin
- Overhanging swelling (lobules)
- Deep cracks in the skin or skin folds

Individuals who treat their lymphedema early and continue to do self-management are less likely to have one of the many potential chronic skin changes seen in long-standing untreated lymphedema.

LIVING WITH LYMPHEDEMA

"The way I think about skin care is that I treat my skin like it's baby skin. Even if it looks fine, I make sure I moisturize it and clean it. Even if you nick it or get an infection, it will be worse if it wasn't protected. You have to be preventive."

Skin Care Strategies

Here are some important ways to protect your skin and prevent infections:

- Prevent dry skin by using moisturizer after bathing; if the lymphedema is in your hands or arms, use moisturizer after washing your hands.

- Prevent cuts and bruises in the skin by using protective gloves or equipment if you are engaging in high-risk activities.

- Use insect repellent or long-sleeved shirts and pants if you are going to be out at night or are at risk of an insect bite.

- Use sunscreen if your skin will be exposed to the sun.

- For lymphedema in the legs, wear footwear at all times when outdoors, especially at the beach. In a pool, water shoes should be worn to prevent injury (such as the skin cracking on the bottom of your feet) from the rough pool floor.

- If you need to shave any lymphatic areas, use an electric razor; a razor blade can cut the skin. You can use an electric razor on your head, neck, face, armpits, back, bikini area or legs.

- Avoid hair-removal treatments involving waxing; the heat from wax can damage the skin and remove the top layer of skin. Threading would be a safer alternative.

- Avoid chemical hair removers, as these can be very harsh and can alter the normal pH of the skin or dry out the skin.

- Avoid skin punctures, such as blood draws or needles, in the lymphedema limb, as these could damage the skin and allow bacteria to enter the body.

- If you have lymphedema in your hand or arm, use gloves when doing housework, gardening, dishes, car repairs or any tasks that could cut your skin or that involve immersing your hands in water or chemical solutions for a prolonged period of time.

- For arm and leg lymphedema, avoid cutting the cuticle (the skin around the nails), as this will damage the skin and can introduce bacteria into the body.

- For those with head and neck lymphedema, make sure you use shampoos and conditioners with the proper pH level, in the range of 4 to 6. Hair dyes have never been reported on in the literature, but these could potentially dry out the scalp and cause irritation to the skin on the head and neck. Make sure you use a licensed barber or hairdresser who cleans their tools appropriately and uses the appropriate products on your hair.

- Treat fungal nail infections (these usually occur on the toenails) with prescription topical creams or ointments.

- Be careful around pets that might scratch or bite.

HOW TO: Protect Your Skin While Washing Your Hands and Showering

1. Wash with a cleanser that has a pH level between 4 to 6.

2. Do not use washcloths, sponges, scrubbing brushes, puffs or loofahs to remove dirt or dead/dry skin; this abrasiveness can damage the skin's barrier. Let dry skin fall off naturally.

3. Do not use very hot water, as this can dry the skin and increase circulation of blood and lymphatic fluid to the lymphedema limb.

4. Make sure to rinse well and remove all the soap/cleanser.

5. Pat the skin dry with a towel (do not rub it dry).

6. Make sure to properly dry out creases, skin folds and the areas between the fingers and toes. For tight swollen spaces, cotton balls or Q-tips can be very helpful. Meticulously drying the skin can prevent tiny cuts from developing in moist areas, such as between the toes.

7. Apply a pH-appropriate lotion or moisturizer to your skin after using water on the lymphedema limb.

The Bottom Line

Skin care is one of the key elements of complete decongestive therapy (CDT), which is the gold standard of care for lymphedema. Proper skin care for lymphedema includes choosing lotions and cleansers with a pH level between 4 and 6; preventing bug bites, scratches, sunburns and other injuries; using an electric razor if you shave; and seeking immediate medical attention for infections. Remember, prevention is key! Be sure to discuss specific strategies for your unique needs with your lymphedema therapist. Be vigilant and stay safe.

CHAPTER 4

Manual Lymphatic Drainage

Manual lymphatic drainage, also known as MLD, is a gentle skin-stretching technique used in a progressive and logical way to stimulate the lymphatic system and increase the rate at which lymphatic fluid is removed from a swollen area. Many experts believe it is one of the key components of lymphedema treatment and recovery. Some people consider MLD to be similar to massage, but it is, in fact, not a massage technique — massage therapy targets deep tissues and muscles and uses more pressure than MLD.

The motions and techniques used in MLD are just light pressure movements. The goal is to use enough pressure to get maximum skin stretch but not enough pressure to feel the muscles or tendons. These movements, also known as strokes, are done in the direction of the desired fluid movement. They are used to activate the smooth muscles in the lymphatic vessels, which, in turn, triggers a faster rate of opening and closing of the lymphatic channels. This causes lymphatic fluid to move through the lymphatic system at a faster rate.

The pressure used in this technique is gentle; if you were to put this amount of pressure on your eyeball, you would feel no discomfort. If you have been through the intensive phase of treatment, you may already understand the level of pressure needed for this technique. Too much pressure — like the pressure used in deep-tissue massage — can temporarily damage the lymphatic vessels that lie just below the skin's surface.

In MLD, 10 to 15 strokes are applied to the same area to maximize the rate of fluid movement from an area, before moving on to the next area. There is a pause between each stroke to allow the tissue to come back to its resting position. This pause is important because the lymphatic fluid needs to move through the surface lymphatic vessels in the layers of skin.

Your lymphedema therapist will use MLD as part of the intensive phase of your treatment, and you can also benefit during the maintenance phase by performing MLD on yourself. You will typically find the most benefit from a self-MLD session that lasts between 10 and 15 minutes, but more time can be spent on each session if necessary to move more fluid.

The main objective of performing MLD is to reroute the lymphatic fluid by getting it to go around the blocked or damaged areas and find the healthy lymph vessels. Once the lymphatic fluid

LIVING WITH LYMPHEDEMA

"I do MLD every morning when I get up, make it a routine. When I sleep, I am not elevating. It only takes 5 minutes."

DID YOU KNOW?

The intensive phase is the first phase of treatment, when the goal is to reduce the size of the limb as much as possible. The maintenance phase is the second phase of treatment, and the goal is to maintain the reduced size of the limb.

finds its way to the healthy vessels, it can be transported to where it is supposed to go: the large veins at the base of your neck, called the subclavian veins, which return the lymphatic fluid to the bloodstream (just before it enters the heart).

You can think of it like doing a maze, but you begin with the finish line and work your way backward to the starting point and then return to the finish line. Once you have cleared the pathway along the maze, the lymphatic fluid can follow this pathway and get to where it needs to be.

Consult with your lymphedema therapist to plan a pathway, or "roadmap," that is catered to your individual needs and that you can do yourself. When you perform your own MLD after proper training, this is referred to as self-MLD. If you are doing MLD correctly, you are increasing the rate of lymphatic-vessel contractions, which creates a suction-like effect from the lymph nodes, thereby moving the trapped lymphatic fluid. Each body part will have a different roadmap. For example, in right-arm lymphedema (due to breast cancer), the roadmap is: neck, left underarm, across the back from the left underarm to the right underarm (moving fluid to the left underarm), and finally from the right shoulder down to the fingers.

DID YOU KNOW?

The normal rate of the lymphatic system is 5 to 10 contractions per minute. After manual lymphatic drainage, it can go up to 20 to 30 contractions per minute.

Differences between Massage and MLD

MASSAGE	MANUAL LYMPHATIC DRAINAGE
Goal is deep-tissue pressure to realign muscle fibers	Goal is skin stretch to encourage flow of lymphatic fluid
High pressure	Low, gentle pressure
Increases blood flow and lymphatic fluid to the area	Reduces lymphatic fluid accumulation
Treats muscle, joint or tendon injury	Reduces lymphedema
Done by massage therapists, physiotherapists, etc.	Done only by lymphedema therapists

Effects of MLD

The main effects of manual lymphatic drainage include:

- An increase of fluid movement from the spaces between cells (interstitial spaces) into lymphatic vessels and back to the large blood vessels leading to the heart
- A reduction in lymphedema swelling
- An increase in lymphatic-vessel smooth-muscle pumping
- A relaxation effect on the muscles (called a parasympathetic response)
- A reduction in pain

LIVING WITH LYMPHEDEMA

"MLD is part of my morning routine. It has to become a habit, like brushing your teeth in the morning."

A Word of Caution

Consult with your lymphedema therapist before performing MLD if the MLD pathway crosses over an area of cancer spread (metastatic area) or if you have any of the following conditions:

- Congestive heart failure
- Renal failure
- Liver disease
- Acute infection (MLD could spread bacteria)
- Acute deep vein thrombosis (DVT)
- Bronchial asthma (in some cases, MLD could trigger an attack)
- Uncontrolled hyperthyroidism
- Uncontrolled high blood pressure
- Pregnancy (first trimester)

If your lymphedema condition requires that you apply MLD in the deep abdominal area, please consult with your lymphedema therapist before beginning treatment if any of the following applies to you:

- Currently undergoing radiation to the abdominal area or have experienced past radiation to the abdominal area
- Pregnancy (all trimesters)
- Menstruation
- Recent abdominal surgery
- Diverticulosis, Crohn's disease or colitis (digestive issues)
- Aortic aneurysm

Research Review: MLD

In 2015, a research team in India looked at the effect of MLD in comparison to resistance exercise (weight lifting) on lymphedema in postsurgical breast cancer patients. The study divided 20 women with breast-cancer-related lymphedema into two groups: 10 women were treated with MLD, resistance exercises and a compression sleeve, while a second group of 10 women were treated with resistance exercises and a compression sleeve (no MLD). All participants had four therapy sessions per week for 8 weeks. After the intervention, the researchers found that both groups had an improvement in limb-volume reduction, but the group that had the MLD achieved longer-lasting reductions in volume.

In 2017, Shao and colleagues did a systematic review and meta-analysis to determine if adding MLD to standard therapy could manage breast-cancer-related lymphedema more effectively than without it. They found four randomized control trials, totaling 234 patients, and the results showed a significant difference in the reduction in lymphedema when MLD was added to the treatment.

The key, however, is to ensure that MLD is part of an overall lymphedema treatment plan; MLD is inadequate by itself. It is best if it is used as part of complete decongestive therapy, which also includes exercise, skin care and compression.

Below are details on some other key studies on MLD.

STUDY #1

In a 2002 study, Williams conducted a randomized study of MLD in 31 individuals with breast-cancer-related lymphedema in one arm and the trunk. The women were divided into two groups. Group A received 45 minutes of MLD 5 days per week for 3 weeks, received no treatment for 6 weeks, then performed 20 minutes of daily self-MLD for 3 weeks. Group B received the same treatment but in the reverse order, namely: performed self-MLD for 3 weeks, received no treatment for 6 weeks, then received MLD for 5 days per week for 3 weeks.

MLD is inadequate by itself. It is best if it is used as part of complete decongestive therapy, which also includes exercise, skin care and compression.

At the beginning of the study and at weeks 3, 9 and 12, the following details were measured or gathered:

- Arm circumference (every $1\frac{1}{2}$ inches/4 cm up the limb)
- Caliper skin-fold thickness in the trunk (torso)
- Skin thickness (measured with high-frequency skin ultrasound)
- Quality-of-life (QoL) questionnaire
- Symptoms (pain, heaviness, etc.)

At the start of the study, there were no differences between groups A and B. After the study, these results were seen:

GROUP	LIMB-VOLUME REDUCTION	CALIPER SKIN TEST	SKIN THICKNESS	QUALITY OF LIFE	SYMPTOMS
Group A (started with MLD)	$2\frac{1}{2}$ oz (71 mL)	Reduced swelling in trunk after MLD	Reduced skin thickness	Improved QoL scale	Improved pain scores
Group B (started with self-MLD)	1 oz (30 mL)	No change	No change	No change	No change

In summary, this study found that MLD reduced limb volume, upper arm thickness, pain and heaviness, and it increased quality of life. The investigators were able to demonstrate that MLD can work even without bandaging, but they acknowledged that the most comprehensive program is one that combines MLD with compression bandaging, skin care and exercise (complete decongestive therapy, or CDT). The study also suggested that the women in Group A understood how to perform self-MLD better after first having 3 weeks of MLD treatment performed by a professional.

STUDY #2

In 2004, McNeely and a team of researchers from Canada investigated the difference in arm-volume reduction in two groups; Group A used compression bandaging in combination with MLD while Group B used just compression bandaging (no MLD). In total, 50 women with lymphedema were randomly assigned to one of the two research groups, both of which were given 4 weeks of treatment.

GROUP	TREATMENT	REDUCTION IN VOLUME USING WATER DISPLACEMENT	REDUCTION IN VOLUME USING LIMB CIRCUMFERENCE
Group A	Compression bandaging and MLD (five 45-minute sessions per week for 4 weeks)	46%	44%
Group B	Compression bandaging	38%	37%

The key result from this study is that those with mild lymphedema who received both compression bandaging and MLD treatments had a significantly larger reduction in the volume of their lymphedema compared to those who received only compression bandaging. Those with early mild lymphedema had better results than those with chronic lymphedema in both groups, which substantiates that early diagnosis and treatment of lymphedema yield the best outcome.

Self-MLD

The results of MLD can vary depending on the amount of training you receive in self-MLD and the amount of monitoring you have by your lymphedema therapist. The more know-how and training you receive in self-MLD treatment techniques and options, the better your results. There is substantial evidence to show that adopting self-treatment practices for your lymphedema will improve your overall recovery. Although much of the research has focused on people with cancer-related lymphedema, it follows that lymphedema from any cause can benefit from self-MLD. Performing self-MLD can help you feel empowered and improve your lymphedema, and it provides an effective self-treatment when MLD by a professional isn't available or once MLD sessions are completed. Finding a supportive professional will help you optimize your self-management program.

Things to Consider When Doing Self-MLD

- Don't begin self-MLD before receiving all the training from your lymphedema therapist. You need to know how much pressure to apply, your unique pathway and how to perform a proper stroke.

- Perform self-MLD for 10 to 15 minutes at least once per day. (If you have more congestion or more pain, self-MLD can be done as often as needed in a day.)

- Do 10 to 15 strokes for each step in the sequence.

- Spend time doing self-MLD to boost the lymphatic system before exercise or strenuous activities. Opening up your lymphatic pathways before exercise may help prevent congestion from accumulating while you exercise.

- Use your entire hand and not just your fingertips. This is less painful and increases the surface area you are treating with each stroke.

- Use a light pressure to stretch the skin; no redness should be seen on the skin's surface. If you feel muscles or tendons, you're using too much pressure.

- Do not slide over the skin, as this won't produce the desired maximum skin stretch and will create friction and redness in the area.

- Start at the top of the limb and move your way down toward your fingers or toes.

- Never work in an area where lymph nodes have been removed (such as the underarm, or axilla), as those pathways are unable to handle the transport of excess fluid.

What to Avoid

For those with lymphedema in both arms, it is best to do shorter sessions or have someone help you with your self-MLD, because you don't want to overuse either arm, which would increase swelling. For those with lymphedema in one arm but at risk for lymphedema in the other arm, it is very important to listen to your body and only do short self-MLD sessions or have help doing self-MLD.

Avoid straining your shoulder or arm while doing self-MLD, as this could lead to overuse strains in the muscles on your unaffected side. Make sure you are sitting in a comfortable position to avoid straining other areas of the body, such as your back or neck. If you suspect a skin infection (cellulitis), discontinue your self-MLD until you have started antibiotics and your symptoms have started to improve. It is best to get clearance to start self-MLD from your doctor or lymphedema therapist after an infection.

CAUTION

The instructions in the pages that follow are not inclusive of all the strokes, sequences and techniques used by lymphedema therapists. These should be used only in consultation with your therapist who has determined — by assessment — which ones are best for you. Bring this book to your assessment and review which of the techniques are right for you. Your lymphedema therapist may add to, modify or delete some of the steps. These general steps do not replace a lymphedema therapy program or certification and should not be used by untrained or uncertified health-care workers to treat your lymphedema.

Neck Self-MLD Sequence

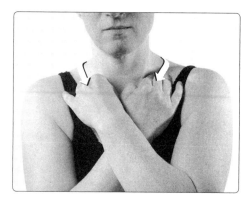 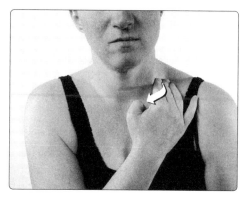

1. The first area to focus on is the spot where all the lymphatics drain into the veins in your neck, which then return it to your heart. It is just above your collarbone in the hollow that would form if you hunched your shoulders forward. The stroke is very light and stretches the skin in a backwards "J" motion (it's a "J" shape when looking down, not in a mirror). Try crossing your hands and using your index and middle fingers to do both sides at the same time or use one hand to do one side at a time. The stroke is down and inward (see arrows). Lift your hand after each stroke to let the skin return to its resting position. Begin with this for all self-MLD.

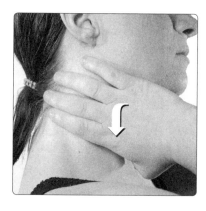

2. Next begin working on the lymphatic pathways along the sides of your neck. Using four flat fingers on the sides of your neck just below your ears, gently stretch the skin back and down (see arrow) and then let it return to its starting place. Depending on the size of your hand and the length of your neck, you may need to divide the neck into two sections to treat your whole neck. You can do both sides of your neck at the same time (uncross your hands) or one side of your neck at a time.

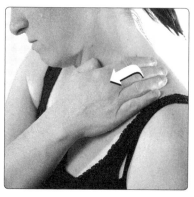

3. The lymphatic pathways on the back of your neck have to travel through your trapezius muscles along the tops of your shoulders between your neck and shoulder joints. This is the muscle that often feels tense on most people. You are going to open up this pathway before working on the back of your neck. It is easiest to do one side at a time for this stroke. Use four flat fingers to gently urge the lymph to come through this muscle to the veins at the front of your neck (see arrow). Imagine the pathways flowing in waves through the muscle and go with the wave. This is a gentle touch (not a deep massage, which most people use for a shoulder rub).

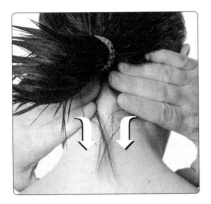

4. To stimulate the lymphatic pathways on the back of your neck, use four flat fingers just below the bony ridge at the back of your skull. Your fingertips do not meet at the spine; rather, leave a little space. Stretch the skin toward the spine in your neck and then downward (see arrows). Let the skin return to its resting position between strokes. Again, you may have to divide the neck into two sections to cover your whole neck.

Source: *Integrated Lymph Drainage. Used with permission.*

Arm Self-MLD Sequence

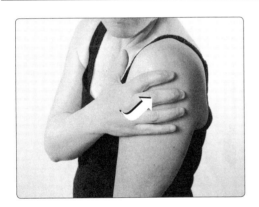 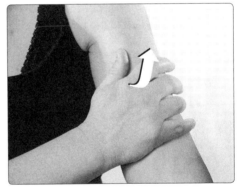

1. *Back of upper arm:* Stroke upward using the entire hand along the side and as far back as you can reach on the upper arm to the area indicated by the arrows. The goal is to direct the fluid around the back of the bony part of the shoulder. Remember that this pathway goes through the trapezius muscle, which you opened in Step 3 of the neck sequence.

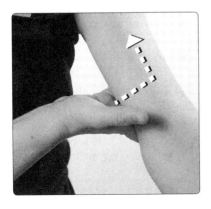

2. The lymphatic fluid in your upper arm usually flows toward the armpit. The alternative pathway we are using sends the fluid to the back of the arm instead. Place your opposite hand on the back of the affected upper arm and stretch the skin in a circular motion toward the back of the arm as indicated by the dotted arrow. As this area softens, slide your hand down the arm toward the elbow and repeat the motion.

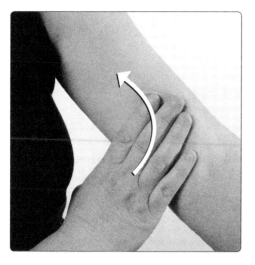

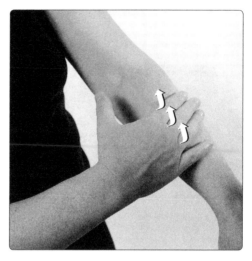

3. To drain the other side of the same upper arm, place your hand on the front of the arm and stretch the skin in a circular motion toward the back of the arm (away from the armpit) as indicated by the arrow. Then repeat Step 1 to bring this fluid up to the neck.

4. *Forearm:* With the palm of your affected arm facing down, use the fingers of your opposite hand to stretch the skin of the forearm in a circular motion toward the upper arm (see arrows).

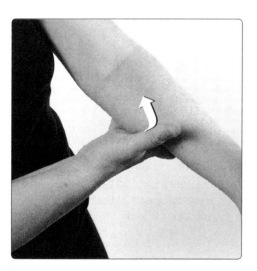

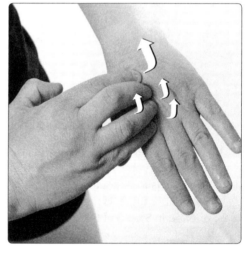

5. Next work on the opposite side of the forearm. Make sure your forearm is in a relaxed position when you work on it.

6. *Hand:* For the hand, using your fingertips, make circling strokes with your fingertips to send the fluid in the direction of the larger arrow. Between your knuckles is a place that fluid can easily collect. To clear this, use your fingertips between the bones of the knuckles and gently circle toward the wrist, as is shown by the small arrows.

Source: *Integrated Lymph Drainage. Used with permission.*

Leg Self-MLD Sequence

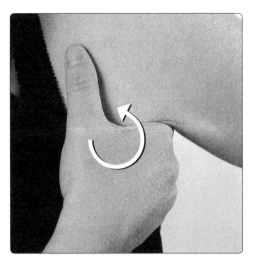

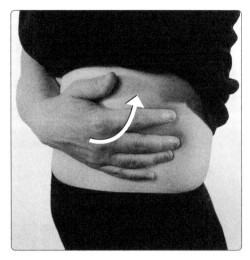

1. *Armpit:* After doing the neck sequence, you are going to stimulate the lymph nodes in the armpit of the affected side. To do this, place the hand of your opposite arm into your armpit with four flat fingers. The direction of the circle is into the armpit and then upward toward the neck (see arrow). Remember to pause briefly between each stroke.

2. *Side:* Along the side of your torso on the affected side, use your entire hand to stroke the skin upward toward the armpit (see arrow), which you have just opened. You could also use the palm of your hand to stretch the skin in a circular way toward the armpit. This gives the leg an alternative pathway to the armpit (instead of trying to go through the nodes at the top of the leg and abdomen).

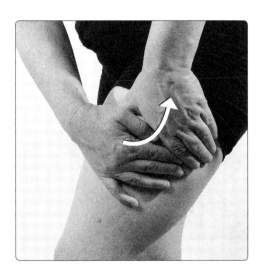

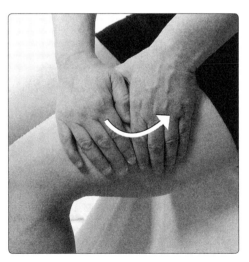

3. *Thigh:* Stroke or make circles with the palms of both hands in the direction shown by the arrows.

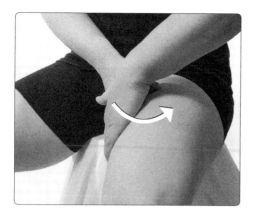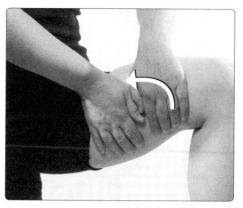

4. With your hands placed flat against the inner thigh, pull the skin toward the top of the thigh (see arrows).

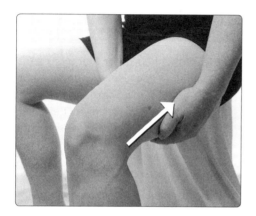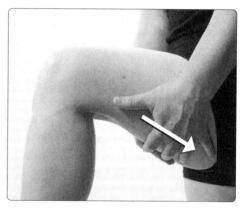

5. With your hands placed under the thigh, pull the skin up toward the buttocks (see arrows).

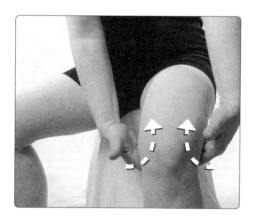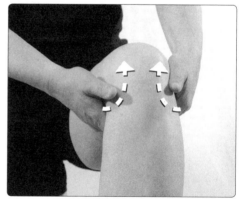

6. *Back of the knee:* To stimulate the nodes and deep pathways behind the knee, place the fingers of both hands behind the knee, with your thumbs lightly resting on the top of the knee. Circle the skin toward the center of the back of the knee and then upward toward the thigh as shown by the dotted arrows.

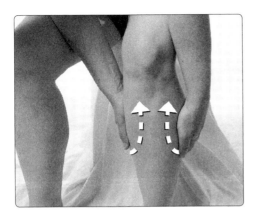 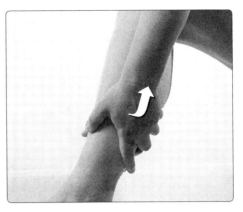

7. *Lower leg:* Stroke the leg upward toward the knee on both the front and back of the calf (see arrows).

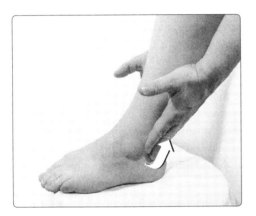 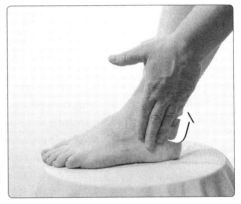

8. *Achilles tendon:* Behind the ankle is a place where fluid likes to collect. To clear this area, place the fingers of both hands on the respective sides of your ankle, behind the ankle bones. Circle the skin upward toward the calf (see arrows). This area may take many repetitions to clear.

Source: Integrated Lymph Drainage. Used with permission.

The Bottom Line

Manual lymphatic drainage is a gentle, systematic technique used to stretch the skin and increase the activity of your healthy lymphatic pathways. It is important to incorporate this technique into your management plan for lymphedema on any part of the body. It plays a vital role in the intensive phase by helping reduce lymphatic volume; in the maintenance phase, it helps stabilize the swelling. Learning self-manual lymphatic drainage to incorporate into your daily home program is essential to taking control of your lymphedema.

> **➡ PRO TIP**
> Maintenance visits with your lymphedema therapist are sometimes required, as self-MLD may not remove all of the swelling. Schedule visits as needed to maintain a stable limb size. Don't be afraid to follow up with your therapist as often as needed.

CHAPTER 5

Multilayer Compression Bandaging

LIVING WITH LYMPHEDEMA

"You've got to learn how to do your wraps [bandaging] yourself. It's important. If you run into trouble and you can't get in to see your therapist, you can wrap it yourself."

Compression bandaging, also called bandaging, multilayer compression bandaging, short-stretch bandaging or wrapping, is one of the most important treatments for lymphedema. It involves three or more layers of bandage material that together provide adequate pressure to a limb to reduce lymphedema. The bandaging must be done in such a way as to produce and maintain the normal pressure gradient of the limb.

Bandaging is the most effective tool to reduce limb volume and can be used in many situations. It is used in the active stage of treatment, also called the intensive phase, when the largest limb-volume reduction is usually possible. It can also be used to maintain the volume reduction that a lymphedema therapist has achieved after treating a flare-up or whenever you feel you need additional support.

If your lymphedema fluctuates significantly while wearing your compression garments, bandaging can be used every night or every other night to help reduce the volume changes that are occurring during the day. For best results, you should treat your lymphedema early and before dense scar tissue has started to develop. However, even if you have long-standing untreated lymphedema, you will see significant improvements by using multilayer compression bandaging. You can learn to self-bandage with a bit of guidance and practice.

FAQ

Q. How does bandaging work?

A. Bandaging works by applying pressure to a swelled area, which presses the fluid out of the congested tissue into the lymphatic vessel. It also reduces leakage from the circulatory system, which means less additional pooling of lymphatic fluid.

Research Review: Multilayer Compression Bandaging

There has been a lot of research done on multilayer compression bandaging and its benefits for lymphedema.

STUDY #1

A Swedish study conducted in 1999 examined 38 female patients with arm lymphedema after breast cancer treatment that included lymph node removal. For the first part of the study, all participants received short-stretch compression bandaging for 2 weeks. Bandages were changed every 2 days. In the first 2 weeks, everyone benefited — the volume of the arm reduced by an average of 6.4 ounces (188 mL), or 26%. The participants were then divided into two groups. The first group continued to receive short-stretch compression bandaging and the second group received this treatment as well as daily MLD. The second group experienced a further 1.6-ounce (47 mL) reduction (11%), compared to a 0.67-ounce (20 mL) reduction (4%) in the first group (bandaging only, no MLD). All the women reported less heaviness and tension in the arm, and the women who had short-stretch compression bandaging plus MLD also had a significant reduction in pain.

Cited in this study was a similar study, conducted previously by Johansson and colleagues, that achieved a 60% volume reduction with bandaging, MLD and exercise combined (MLD alone showed a reduction of only 15% in volume).

STUDY #2

This study was authored by Myrna King and colleagues in 2011 and examined whether a compression garment or compression bandaging was more effective as an initial treatment strategy for women with breast-cancer-related lymphedema. Twenty-one women were divided into two groups; both groups had complete decongestive therapy (CDT), but the first group used bandaging and the second group used custom-made compression sleeves.

GROUP	CDT TREATMENT PLAN	VOLUME REDUCTION AT 10 DAYS	VOLUME REDUCTION AT 3 MONTHS
Bandaging group	• Manual lymph drainage • Skin care • Exercise • 3-layer compression bandaging	2.37 oz (70 mL)	3.29 oz (97.5 mL)
Compression sleeve group	• Manual lymph drainage • Skin care • Exercise • Compression sleeve	0.17 oz (5 mL)	1.69 oz (50 mL)
Difference		2.2 oz (65 mL)	1.6 oz (47.5 mL)

LIVING WITH LYMPHEDEMA

"I was very intimidated with the wrapping. I was drawn to the nice-looking sleeves; they were so cool. When my therapist suggested wrapping, I was intimidated. It took several weeks. I would do it in front of my therapist and she would correct me. I'm doing it with my eyes shut now."

➡ PRO TIP

A simple bandage, like the one described starting on page 65, can give you an initial volume reduction. For even more reduction, adding foam can help.

CAUTION

Tensor bandages, or bandages used in sports injuries, stretch too much and should not be used in lymphedema. The elastic in them can make lymphedema worse.

The results are clear: the bandaging group lost almost 50% more fluid volume than the compression sleeve group. The results of this study coincide with results observed in clinical settings. Although the study involved individuals undergoing daily treatments, similar results can be seen with just three treatments per week, though it may take longer. If you can master the skill of doing your own manual lymphatic drainage and bandaging, you can help your lymphedema therapist during the intensive phase of treatment and achieve similar results (this may not be true if your case is more complicated).

STUDY #3

The above results are similar to a study published by Badger and colleagues in 2000. In this study, 90 patients with arm lymphedema were divided into two groups. Both groups received manual lymphatic drainage (MLD), exercise and skin care for the first 18 days. But one group also did compression bandaging every day for those 18 days. After the 18 days, both groups wore a compression sleeve for 6 months. The group that received compression bandaging prior to switching to the sleeve experienced a 50% greater reduction in their lymphedema.

Bandaging Supplies

The type of bandaging material you use is critical to achieving the best results. Short-stretch bandages are special bandages that have very little stretch to them and are specifically designed to treat lymphedema. Lymphedema bandages can be found wherever you purchase your compression garments, from your lymphedema therapist or from online stores (see Resources, page 258). There are many bandage brands on the market, so it is best to make sure that the product you are using is designed for lymphedema.

If your lymphedema has hardened, you will need additional materials under the bandaging to achieve the best results. Some of these materials are open-cell or closed-cell foams, channel foams, gray foams, white foams and chip pads. You can purchase many of these products through lymphedema supply stores or online.

It is best to speak with your lymphedema therapist to determine which bandaging techniques and products should be used for your lymphedema. Lymphedema therapists will often try different bandaging materials to make sure they are working effectively and not causing any new issues. Bandages that are applied incorrectly can result in wounds or other problems.

Once the correct bandaging technique is determined, you can then be taught how to safely put on your own bandages. At this point, you and your therapist can work in partnership: you can bandage on days that you don't attend the clinic, and your therapist can perform MLD and bandaging on your clinic days. Your lymphedema therapist can also show you how to make adjustments to your bandages if they slip, which often happens as the volume reduces. This partnership will help you achieve the best results.

The table below provides a summary of some products that are currently available for your bandaging needs. Check with your lymphedema therapist for the options that will work best for your particular needs. There are many different manufacturers for the different products, so check what is easily accessible where you live.

Bandaging Materials

BANDAGES	MATERIAL	SIZE	PURPOSE	BRANDS (MANUFACTURER)
Gauze bandages for fingers and toes	Cotton with elastic Simple first aid gauze with elastic can also be used	Rolls are 13 feet (4 m) long and come in the following widths: Fingers: 2½ inches (6 cm) Toes: 1½ inches (4 cm)	Compresses toes and fingers	Elastomull (BSN) Mollelast (Lohmann & Rauscher)
Stockinette or tubular bandage	Cotton	Different sizes are available to treat limbs of all sizes	Protects the skin Absorbs sweat, dead skin, oils Keeps synthetic padding clean	TG (Lohmann & Rauscher) Tricofix (BSN)
Synthetic padding	Synthetic material	Rolls are 10 feet (3 m) long and come in the following widths: Arm or lower leg: 4 inches (10 cm) Thigh or upper leg: 6 inches (15 cm)	Helps evenly distribute pressure from short-stretch bandages Provides comfort for longer wear times	Cellona (Lohmann & Rauscher) Artiflex (BSN)
Short-stretch bandages	Cotton woven together with elastic to get 60% stretch	Rolls are 16 feet (5 m) long and come in the following widths: 1½ inches (4 cm) 2½ inches (6 cm) 3 inches (8 cm) 4 inches (10 cm) 5 inches (12 cm)	Provides compression Moves the lymphatic fluid out of the swollen area, especially when moving or exercising	Comprilan (BSN) Rosidal K (Lohmann & Rauscher)
Open-cell foam	Foam	16 feet by 4 inches (5 m by 10 cm)	Adds additional pressure	CompriFoam (BSN)
Closed-cell foam	Foam	Different sizes are available to fit small areas, such as behind the ankle	Adds additional pressure	JobstFoam (BSN) Komprex Foam (Lohmann & Rauscher)
Gray foam or channel foam	Foam	Each sheet 1 foot by 3 feet (30 by 90 cm) and can be cut into ½- or 1-inch (1 or 2.5 cm) thickness	Breaks up scar tissue	Gray foam or Farrow Wrap (Farrow) or channel foam (various)

Learning to Bandage

The technique of bandaging your limb is best explained and demonstrated by your lymphedema therapist; the exact procedure will depend on you and your lymphedema. When you visit your therapist, it is important to bring a support person with you, such as a family member or a friend, so that they can assist you in the first few days of bandaging. It will take several practices before you can put your bandages on by yourself.

Self-bandaging will be much easier to learn when your nondominant arm has the lymphedema; however, with practice, either arm will become easy to bandage. If you have the flexibility to touch your toes and have adequate movement of the hip and knee joints, you will be able to bandage your own legs. If you have a large abdomen or another issue that makes bending over difficult, you will need help bandaging your lower legs.

Ann's Clinical Experience

Bandaging can be used to reduce the swelling in any area of the body; however, in my practice, I use it most often for arm and leg lymphedema. Typically, I introduce bandaging to clients who have two limbs with lymphedema or clients with one limb that is $1\frac{1}{5}$ inches (3 cm) larger in diameter in three or more consecutive spots compared to the unaffected limb. Some of my clients have benefited from chest wall bandaging to reduce swelling after a mastectomy or lumpectomy.

CAUTION

The instructions on the following pages should be used only as a guide to support you when you are in the maintenance phase of treatment and to refresh your memory after you have been taught by your lymphedema therapist. You may not be able to use compression bandaging. Consult with your lymphedema therapist to make sure it is safe for you. (See "A Word of Caution" on page 50.)

How to Put On Compression Bandages: Arm Lymphedema

You Will Need

- Gauze: 2½ inches (6 cm)
- Tubular stockinette with no elastic
- Synthetic padding: 4 inches (10 cm)
- Two or 3 short-stretch washable compression bandages; you'll need at least
  - One 2½-inch (6 cm) bandage
  - One 3-inch (8 cm) bandage
  - One 4-inch (10 cm) bandage (optional, depending on the size of your arm)
- Masking tape
- Scissors

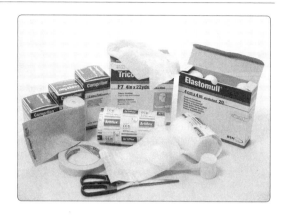

> ⮕ **PRO TIP**
>
> Medical tape can be used but it can be costly and tends to leave a sticky residue on the bandages that will look dirty after a few weeks of use. Use a good-quality brand of masking tape, one that is reasonably priced, leaves no residue, is easy to remove and is readily available in your area.

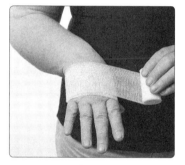

1. Take the 2½-inch (6 cm) gauze roll and wrap it around the hand once. There should be very little to no pull in the bandage.

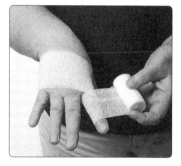

2. Wrap the gauze around the finger twice with 50% stretch.

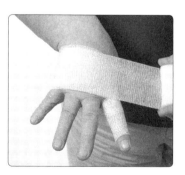

3. Continue around the hand once with the gauze.

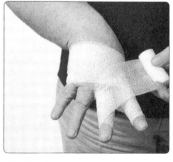

4. Continue around the second finger twice. Continue around the hand once again.

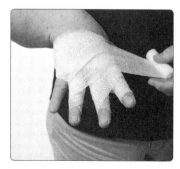

5. Continue around the third finger twice. Continue around the hand once again.

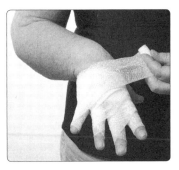

6. Continue around the fourth finger twice and then around the back of the hand to the base of the thumb.

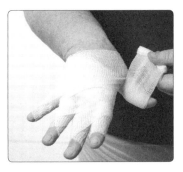

7. Continue around the thumb twice.

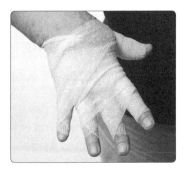

8. Continue wrapping around the hand until the gauze is used up, then use masking tape to secure the end of the gauze.

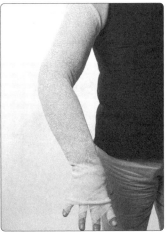

9. Pull your stockinette up over your hand and arm, up to your shoulder.

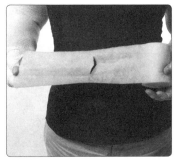

10. Take your synthetic padding (4 inches/10 cm) and cut a hole in it about 7 inches (18 cm) from the end. This is where your thumb will go.

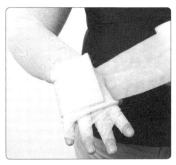

11. Put your thumb through the hole in the synthetic padding and wrap the loose end around the back of your hand.

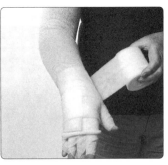

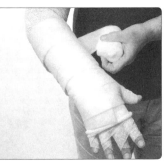

12. Unroll the synthetic padding up your arm, overlapping 50% and with no stretch or pull on the synthetic padding. No pressure should come from the synthetic padding; this is simply a protective layer for the skin that evenly distributes the pressure of the bandages.

⇒ **PRO TIP**

It is not necessary to pull the padding tight; it shouldn't provide any pressure. Padding is used to provide protection to the skin from the bandages, to provide comfort and to help evenly distribute the pressure from the bandages. There are many kinds of padding materials on the market, such as cotton, foam, synthetic or felt.

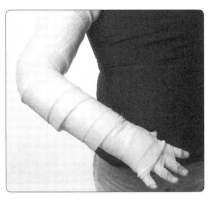

13. This is what the full-arm synthetic padding should look like.

OPTIONAL FOAM

If you have thick, dense or hardened areas of lymphedema, speak to your lymphedema therapist about whether or not foam options should be added to the process after step 13. This is a more advanced technique that depends on individual cases.

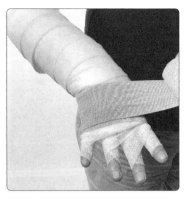

14. Take a 2½-inch (6 cm) short-stretch bandage and wrap it, with 50% stretch, around the hand twice. Start above where the fingers meet the hand.

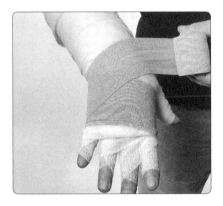

15. From the outside border of the hand across the back of the hand, wrap up to the wrist and go around the wrist to the outside border.

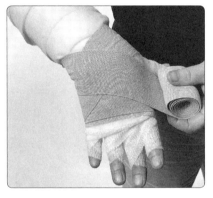

16. Wrap across the back of the hand and down to the inside border of the hand. You will end up back at the outside border of the wrist, with an "X" on the inside of the palm of the hand and an "X" on the back of the hand, like a figure eight.

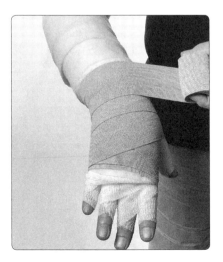

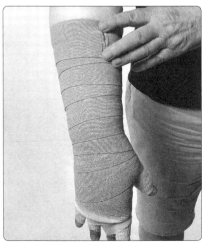

17. Wrap around your wrist, overlapping 50% with 50% stretch in the bandage, until that bandage is completely used up. Tape the end with masking tape.

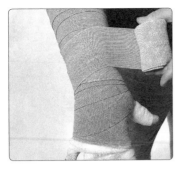 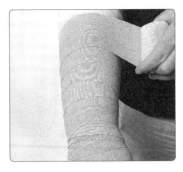

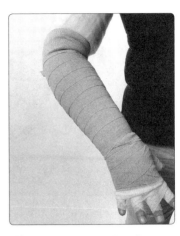

18. Take a 3-inch (8 cm) short-stretch bandage and start at the wrist. Wrap around the wrist, overlapping 50% with 50% stretch, going up the arm. Your elbow should be slightly bent as you go over it. (Overlapping the ends of the bandages ensures even pressure and a proper pressure gradient.)

19. This bandage will end at or above the elbow. Tape the end with masking tape.

> **→ PRO TIP**
>
> If you have short arms, you might achieve enough pressure with just two bandages.

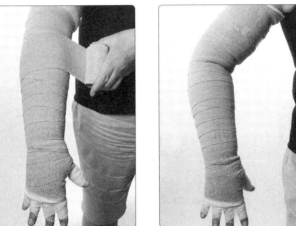 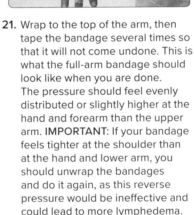

20. If needed, take a 4-inch (10 cm) short-stretch bandage and start just below the elbow, overlapping it 50% with 50% stretch, going up the arm.

21. Wrap to the top of the arm, then tape the bandage several times so that it will not come undone. This is what the full-arm bandage should look like when you are done. The pressure should feel evenly distributed or slightly higher at the hand and forearm than the upper arm. **IMPORTANT:** If your bandage feels tighter at the shoulder than at the hand and lower arm, you should unwrap the bandages and do it again, as this reverse pressure would be ineffective and could lead to more lymphedema.

> **→ PRO TIP**
>
> If you have very swollen or longer arms, and this causes you to run out of bandage, a 4-inch (10 cm) bandage can be applied starting from below the elbow and working your way up to 1 inch (2.5 cm) below the armpit. This should provide comfortable and pain-free pressure to the arm. Your fingers should not turn blue or red or feel cold, painful or numb.

CAUTION

If you have a wound in the area of your lymphedema, before bandaging, consult a wound-care specialist or lymphedema therapist who is familiar with wound-care management. Applying too much pressure or an uneven pressure can worsen wounds and lead to further complications. Having a wound in the area of your lymphedema means your situation is an extremely complex one and your care goes beyond the scope of this book, which is designed for self-management of uncomplicated cases of lymphedema.

How to Put On Compression Bandages: Leg Lymphedema

You Will Need

- Tubular stockinette with no elastic
- Gauze: 1½ inches (4 cm)
- Synthetic padding: one 4-inch (10 cm) and one or two 6-inch (15 cm) paddings
- Short-stretch washable compression bandages; you'll need one 3-inch (8 cm) bandage, two 4-inch (10 cm) bandages and one 5-inch (12 cm) bandage; depending on the size of your leg, more bandages may be needed
- Masking tape
- Scissors

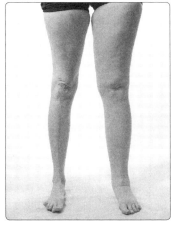

1. This photo shows leg lymphedema prior to bandaging.

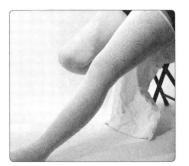

2. Pull your stockinette up to the top of your leg, with the stockinette still extending past your toes. Pull up the stockinette to reveal your foot.

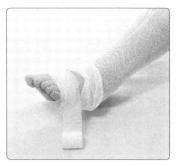

3. Take a 1½-inch (4 cm) gauze roll and wrap it around the foot once with light pressure; do not pull it tight.

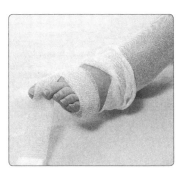

4. Bring the gauze to the base of the big toe and wrap it around the big toe twice, with 50% stretch in the gauze. It should not be pulled so tight that it hurts or the toe changes color.

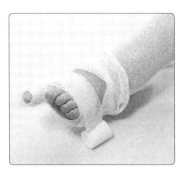

5. Wrap the gauze around the foot once.

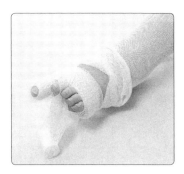

6. Bring the gauze to the base of the second toe and wrap around that toe twice.

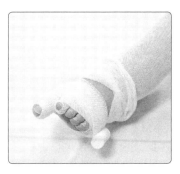

7. Wrap the gauze around the foot once.

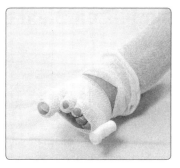

8. Bring the gauze to the base of the third toe and wrap around that toe twice.

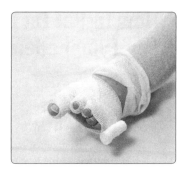

9. Wrap the gauze around the foot once.

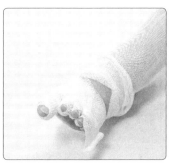

10. Bring the gauze to the base of the fourth toe and wrap around that toe twice.

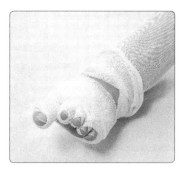

11. Wrap the gauze around the foot once.

➡ PRO TIP

If you have space between your fourth and fifth toes and the area is swollen, then wrap the gauze around the fifth (baby) toe twice and then around the foot one more time. Some people have a very short or curled fifth toe, which makes gauzing around it impossible without the gauze bunching up.

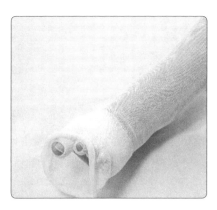

12. Pull the stockinette down over your gauze foot and toes.

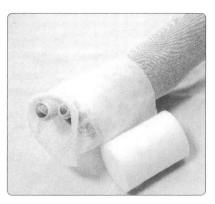

13. Take the small roll of synthetic padding (4 inches/10 cm) and, with the roll facing up, wrap it around the foot one time, starting where the toes meet the foot.

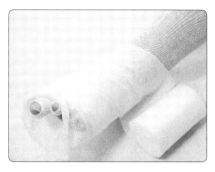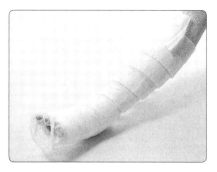

14. Wrap it around the foot and leg, overlapping 50%, until the synthetic padding roll is completely used up. Do not pull it tight. There should be no pressure; rather, its job is to protect the skin and also evenly distribute the pressure of the bandages.

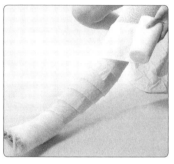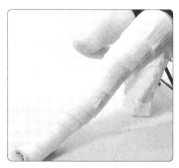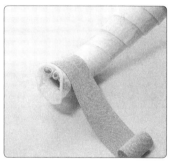

15. Start the larger roll of synthetic padding (6 inches/15 cm) where the last roll ended and overlap 50% up the leg until the roll is used up. If you run out before you reach the top of the leg (this can happen if you have long legs or lots of swelling), three rolls may be needed; begin where the last roll ended and cut the roll when you have covered the full leg.

16. Take the 3-inch (8 cm) short-stretch bandage and start where the toes meet the foot, which should be over the start of the synthetic padding. Wrap it around the foot twice, pulling with 50% stretch.

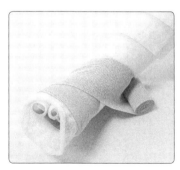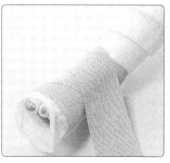

17. Bring the bandage across the top of the ankle and foot, with the foot flexed up toward you (it's easier to wrap if the foot is at 90 degrees).

18. Continue around the back of the ankle and over the top of the foot; the bandages should resemble an "X" pattern.

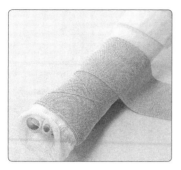

19. Continue around the heel and over the top of the ankle again.

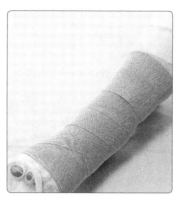
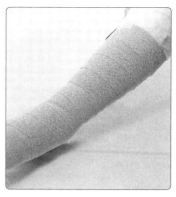

20. Continue to wrap the bandage, overlapping 50% with 50% stretch, up the leg until the first bandage is used up. Tape the end with masking tape.

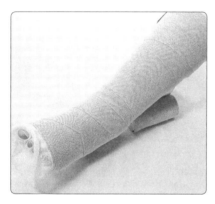
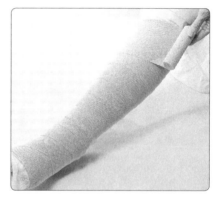

21. Take the second short-stretch bandage (4 inches/10 cm) and start it just above the ankle crease, overlapping 50% with 50% stretch. Unwrap the bandage up the leg until it ends around the knee or slightly above (the knee should be slightly bent). Tape the end with masking tape.

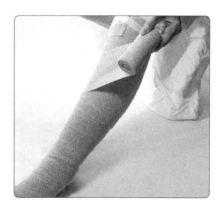
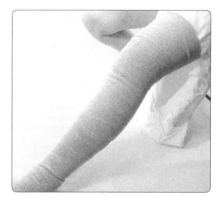

22. Take another 4-inch (10 cm) short-stretch bandage and start that below the knee. Unwrap the bandage, overlapping 50% with 50% stretch, up the leg until it is used up.

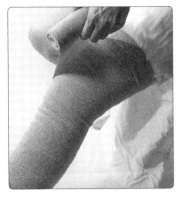 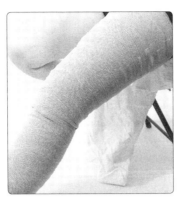

23. Take the final and widest short-stretch bandage (5 inches/ 12 cm) and start that just above the knee. Unwrap the bandage, overlapping 50% with 50% stretch, up the leg to the groin.

⟶ **PRO TIP**

The reason we overlap the short-stretch bandages is because there is reduced pressure at the end of the bandage. The overlapping helps to create a pressure gradient from the hand or foot up to the shoulder or hip.

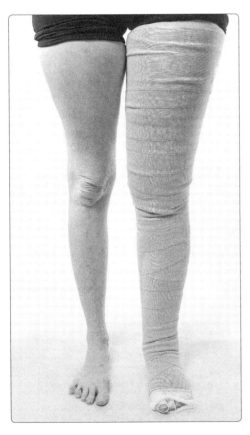

24. This is what the full-leg bandage should look like when you are done.

Checklist for Bandaging

☐ Limb function (your bandaged limb should still be able to function and should not be too restricted)

☐ Range of motion (the joint under the bandage should still have full range of motion; for example, you should be able to move your shoulder and elbow, or your knee and hip)

☐ Comfort

☐ Support

☐ Shoes stay on (you should be able to walk without your shoes slipping off; this reduces the risk of falls; try large shoes, Crocs, wide shoes, cast shoes or sandals with Velcro toe and heel straps)

☐ No pain

☐ No discomfort

☐ No discoloration in fingers or toes

LIVING WITH LYMPHEDEMA

"I don't mix my lymphedema wraps with my other laundry, since I've had cellulitis a couple of times out of the blue (I had a fever and blotchy skin). I wash them inside a mesh bag and in warm water, and I hang them up; I don't put them in the dryer."

Washing Your Bandaging Supplies

This section outlines tips and techniques for taking care of your bandages, which will help them last longer and save you money. Some bandages can be washed in the machine, some need to be hand-washed, and others can't be washed at all. If your bandages are heavily soiled (and can handle the washing machine; see below for specifics), you can machine-wash. Otherwise, wash by hand, since machine-washing will shorten the life of your bandages. Instructions for both types of washing can be found below.

Gauze Finger/Toe Bandages

- Wash after each use.
- Can be hand-washed if done carefully.
- Hang to dry.
- Replace after one or two uses.

Stockinettes

- Wash after each use.
- Can be machine-washed in a linen bag with your short-stretch bandages. Alternatively, you can hand-wash them.
- Hang to dry.
- Replace them when they become misshapen or stretched out, or if they develop holes.

Synthetic Padding

- According to the manufacturers, these should be hand-washed and are not machine-washable; however, some people have had success machine-washing them in a linen bag and laying them flat or hanging them to dry.
- Replace them when they become too thin or dirty.

Foam

- These are not washable in the machine or by hand.
- Replace when they start to thin out or become too compressed.

HOW TO: Machine-Wash and Dry Bandages

1. Wash your bandages in warm or cold water daily to bring back their stretch (avoid hot water, as this damages the elastic).

2. Do not use chlorine or non-chlorine bleach or fabric softener.

3. Lay bandages flat to dry, as hand-wringing, machine-drying and hanging to dry will cause the wet elastic to stretch.

HOW TO: Hand-Wash and Dry Bandages

1. Make sure your sink is clean before beginning.

2. Fill sink with warm water and only a drop or two of mild liquid soap, such as dish soap or laundry soap. (Some bandage manufacturers make special washing solutions that you can purchase from your bandaging supply store.)

3. Put bandages in the soapy water and stir them around for a few minutes.

4. Drain soapy water.

5. Refill sink with clean warm water to rinse, and repeat this process three times to make sure all the soap is rinsed from the bandages.

6. Lay the bandages out on a clean, dry bath towel and roll them up in the towel to remove as much water as possible.

7. Lay bandages flat on another clean, dry bath towel to dry. This can be done over a heating vent.

8. Once dry, roll the bandages up as they were when you first purchased them (do not iron).

9. Do not put bandages in the dryer or lay out bandages in direct sunlight.

The Bottom Line

Learning how to bandage your lymphedema is an important skill that is well worth your time and effort to learn. You may feel that you will never master bandaging or that it is too cumbersome and time-consuming, or you may prefer to just put on your compressive sleeve or stocking and head out the door. But learning to bandage will give you independence in managing your lymphedema: you will be able to respond to sudden flare-ups, prepare for flights, and respond to the effects of hot, humid days and many other scenarios when it's not possible to see your lymphedema therapist right away. Although it will take some time to learn, if you persist, soon you will be able to bandage with your eyes closed.

Compression Garments

Compression garments may be the best known of the lymphedema treatments. They're now available in so many more patterns and colors than in years past, and they're becoming a way for you to express your personality through the colors and patterns you choose to wear. You may choose a garment to match your skin tone or you might want to be bold and choose a bright color, such as fuchsia, to proudly wear on your arm or leg. Having color options may make it more appealing for you to wear a compression garment. The garments are available for all shapes, sizes and body types.

What Are Compression Garments?

Compression garments are designed to provide compression, or pressure, to prevent swelling. They are made of fabric that is woven together to form stockings, sleeves, gloves and other apparel. The major manufacturers are in the United States and Germany, and they have many different options available. These garments are a vital component of complete decongestive therapy (CDT) and are used after the intensive phase of treatment has been completed. Garments are a primary part of the maintenance phase and are designed to support the lymphatic system.

If you are in the early stages of lymphedema, such as stage 0 or stage 1 (see page 24 for the stages of lymphedema), you can likely skip the intensive phase with bandaging and go directly to a compression garment to manage your lymphedema. If pitting edema exists, bandaging should be used first to remove the lymphatic fluid, and then a garment can be used.

Compression garments help maintain limb size, but they lead to only a small decrease in circumference, such as $\frac{1}{2}$ to 1 inch (1 to 2.5 cm).

Using Compression Garments as a Preventive Measure

You may not have lymphedema yet but be at a high risk of developing it — for example, if you are scheduled to have more than 10 lymph nodes removed or to undergo radiation treatment, or if you are overweight. In addition to these high-risk conditions, certain activities could further increase your risk, such as exercise, air travel or strenuous and repetitive activities. In these cases, a compression garment can be worn as a preventive measure to reduce your chances of developing lymphedema. Speak with your lymphedema therapist to determine if you should use compression as part of your prevention strategy.

Types of Compression Garments

There are two categories of compression garments: circular knit and flat knit. The type of garment used depends on the stage of lymphedema, the shape of the limb, the quality of the skin and the ease of use.

Considerations When Choosing Compression Garments

CIRCULAR KNIT	FLAT KNIT
Can be purchased over-the-counter	Must be custom-made
Lower cost	Higher cost
No seams	Seams
More stretch	Less stretch
Available in pressure ranges (mm Hg): • 15–20 • 20–30 • 30–40 • 40–50	Available in pressure ranges (mm Hg): • 15–20 • 20–30 • 30–40 • 40–50
Designed for regularly shaped limbs (cone shape) Unable to conform to lobules or limited ability to conform to lobules	Can be customized to fit lobules, creases and irregularly shaped limbs
Available in many colors, styles and patterns	Available in many colors, styles and patterns

If you have an irregularly shaped limb, lobules or creases, or if you have a soft larger thigh or upper arm, a circular knit garment *cannot* be used. This is because the circular knit fabric does not have enough rigidity and will roll up or slip into the creases, creating a tourniquet that will cut off lymphatic flow and blood flow. It could also make the swelling worse or create wounds on the skin. In these cases, it is crucial to use only flat knit garments, which have more rigidity, will not roll and can be designed to fit any shape. It's important that the flat knit garment fits snugly and is the correct length. If it isn't snug enough or is too long, the fabric can slip and bunch up behind the joint, such as at the elbow, knee or ankle.

You should be assessed by a lymphedema garment fitter and lymphedema therapist to determine the best compression prescription for your needs. For example, you may need to use silk pads to protect sensitive areas, such as behind the knee or the front of the elbow. Zippers can be sewn into custom garments to make them easier to put on. Pockets for foam pads can be added to areas where fluid accumulates, such as behind the ankle or on the back of the hand. Typically, custom-made garments can be made with a myriad of options to suit your individual needs.

Arm and Leg Sleeves for Daytime Use

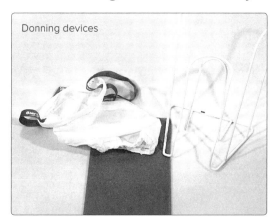

Donning devices

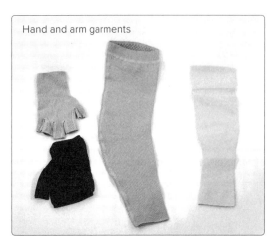

Hand and arm garments

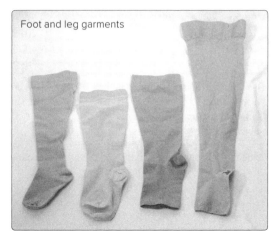

Foot and leg garments

Special Considerations for Older Adults with Lower Leg Lymphedema

If you are over 50 years old and have lower leg lymphedema, it is important for your therapist or fitter to assess the ankle brachial pressure index when deciding which class of compression garment is best for you. (In North America, the index is referred to as ABI; in the United Kingdom, it's ABPI.) You may have some arterial insufficiency in the area, which means your circulation is limited. A Doppler ultrasound should be done to assess the arteries. This chart shows you the level of compression you need based on the results of your ankle-brachial pressure index testing.

ABI Ranges vs. Compression Class

ABI Range	Compression Class for Stockings
>0.8	34–46 mm Hg
0.5–0.8	up to 21 mm Hg
<0.5	Don't use compression stockings; consult a vascular surgeon

Source: *Template for Practice: Compression Hosiery in Lymphedema, International Lymphedema Framework, 2006.*

Fitting for Compression Garments

It is very important that you consult only professionals who have the necessary training to measure and fit you with your lymphedema compression garments. These specialists are called certified compression fitters ("fitters" for short) and have been trained by the manufacturers of compression garments to properly measure and fit their products. Fitters can be lymphedema therapists, health-care professionals or laypeople with specialized training in the measuring and fitting of compression garments. Connecting with a properly trained and skilled fitter is an essential component of your lymphedema treatment.

Compression Prescription

Your lymphedema therapist and your garment fitter should determine what kind of compression garment will work for you, such as the type (for example, knee-high, thigh-high, pantyhose, etc.) and class of compression (for example, 20–30 mm Hg, 30–40 mm Hg, etc.). The type of compression and knit of the garment will be unique to you. The stage of your lymphedema, the shape of your limb, the texture and density of your tissue, your pain level, the quality of your skin,

> ➡ **PRO TIP**
> Garments should be measured once your limb has been maximally reduced with bandaging. Typically, people with lymphedema report that their swelling is the best first thing in the morning, so it is best to be measured for a new compression garment first thing in the morning.

FAQ

Q. Is there any financial support available to help me purchase compression garments?

A. Compression garments can be expensive. Find out from your therapist or fitter what financial support might be available for you. In the United States, your insurance plan may cover the cost of your compression garment, but it depends on the plan you have. In Canada, some private insurance companies cover the cost.

Sometimes government bodies can also help. In Ontario, for example, the government offers the Assistive Devices Program (ADP), which covers 75% of the cost of compression garments for people diagnosed with lymphedema. You must receive a prescription from a specialist recognized by ADP to diagnose lymphedema and purchase your garment from an authorized ADP vendor (an authorized ADP vendor is a store that has a certified fitter approved by the government to fit you for your compression garment). A lymphedema therapist approved by ADP will also need to sign your ADP application.

Connect with your local state or provincial lymphedema association to find out what funding options may be available to you. See Resources, page 257, for more information.

your dexterity, your flexibility and other medical issues you have will all need to be considered when prescribing your compression garment.

Preparing for Your Fitting

Play an active role in selecting your garment type, style and color because you will be the one wearing it.

At the fitting, you should expect that the body part with lymphedema will be exposed, so dress accordingly. The measuring should be done directly on your skin (not over your clothes) to ensure your compression garment properly contours to your limb. Your fitter will take several measurements. Circular knit ready-made garments will require fewer measurements than flat knit custom-made garments. Your fitter should also ask you about your lifestyle, and this will help your fitter select the best product for you.

Play an active role in selecting your garment type, style and color because you will be the one wearing it. Your success in managing your lymphedema is directly related to you wearing your garment as prescribed by your lymphedema therapist.

Once the measurements have been taken, it can take anywhere from 1 week (ready-made) up to 4 weeks (custom-made) for your compression garment to arrive. While you wait, it is important to maintain the reduction you achieved with bandaging, so you must continue to bandage until your new compression garment arrives.

Garments That Stay Up

Another thing to consider when fitting or choosing a garment is how it will stay up and not slip. Here are some options to discuss with your fitter:

- Silicone bands are a good solution and can be added to the top end of a garment.

- Garment glues that are safe to use on skin are available from many garment manufacturers; these add a touch of tackiness, which prevents slipping.

- Some sleeves have shoulder caps with cross-body straps that attach under the other arm; others have bra-strap attachments.

- Some lower-body garments have a waist attachment; it fits like a belt that fastens with Velcro around your waist.

- Full pantyhose are available for when both legs are swollen, or single-leg pantyhose can be used for single-leg lymphedema.

- When both legs are affected and you have difficulty putting on pantyhose, thigh-high stockings can be used with compression bike shorts over top.

FAQ

Q. How often do I need to replace my compression garments?

A. If you are using a garment daily, plan to purchase two garments every 4 to 6 months. You will need two garments because you will need a second garment while you wash your first. If you are very overweight or very active, you may need to renew your garment more often because of the increased wear and tear on the elastic in the garment.

If your garment feels like it is losing its shape, is slipping or is too easy to put on, see your fitter for new garments. The oils from your skin and the residue from skin care products cause a breakdown in the elastic of the fabric.

It is important to keep track of when you purchased your garments and to renew them on time. Too often, people forget to renew their compression garments on time, and when they visit their therapist or fitter, they find out they waited too long and their old garment wasn't working for them anymore, which led to an increase in their lymphedema.

Trying on Your New Garments

When your new garment arrives, try it on with your fitter present. Your fitter should give you instructions for how to put on your garment. Try putting on and taking off your garment on your own; your fitter can address any problems and suggest adjustments. The fitter should assess the fit of the garment to make sure it meets your needs; it should compress the areas where swelling exists and conform to your limb properly.

If you have difficulty putting on your garment by yourself, there are devices available that can help you (see first photo, page 78). When putting on a garment, pull it from the middle of the garment; do not pull it from the end, as this can overstretch the fabric. Use rubber gloves to ensure a good grip on the fabric, and make sure you pull it high enough. Use your gloved hand to run over the fabric several times to even it out and get the creases out. This helps to prevent high-pressure areas.

Do not use lotions prior to putting on your compression garment; petroleum, oils and other ingredients can break down the elastic in the fabric, shortening the lifespan of the compression garment. If you need to use a moisturizer, it's best to put this on before bedtime, when you will not be in your garment for several hours.

FAQ

Q. Why does my swelling increase when I remove my compression garment?

A. Compression garments work by limiting capillary refill; they do not have much of an effect on the protein in the lymph fluid. When you remove your compression garment, the high protein concentration pulls fluid into the tissues, causing rebound swelling. A good strategy is to remove your garment just before you lie down in bed at night. This helps reduce the effect of gravity on rebound swelling.

When to Stop Wearing Your Garment

You should stop wearing your garment if you notice any of the following:

- Redness or rash: If you suspect an infection or have any of the symptoms listed in "Skin Changes with Lymphedema," page 45, seek immediate medical attention.

- Itchiness or sensitivity to the fabric: You may need to be assessed for a possible allergy.

- A bluish color or other discoloration of the limb: This tends to happen in fingers and toes and can be a sign that your garment is too tight.

- Open wounds: The force of putting on a garment will increase the size of the wound.

- A feeling of pins and needles or numbness while wearing your garment: This could mean the garment is too tight or a seam is compressing a nerve.

- An increase in swelling: This indicates that the pressure gradient is not correct.

FAQ

Q. Should I use my compression when I have an infection in my lymphedema limb?

A. It depends. You should not wear your compression when you have an infection if:

- You are not on antibiotics.

- Your limb is very swollen because of the infection. It is likely that your compression garment will not fit properly; if it is too tight, it could damage the initial lymphatics in your skin. Go back to bandaging, as long as it does not cause pain. If the pain is too severe, you may need a few days out of your compression until the antibiotics can take effect and lessen the pain. When that happens, you can bandage or use your garment again.

- Your infection has open skin or a wound. In this case, you will first need proper wound care and bandaging until the skin is healed. It's important to remember that elastic garments will cause a shearing effect on your skin when putting them on, which could open up the skin even more.

You can wear your compression when you have an infection if:

- Your limb isn't very swollen because of the infection.

- You don't have open skin or a wound.

- You have consulted with your doctor or lymphedema therapist and started appropriate and effective antibiotics.

Velcro Compression Garments

→ **PRO TIP**

A typical result when a client uses Velcro compression garments is a 20% reduction in lymphedema.

LIVING WITH LYMPHEDEMA

"I have to wear my compression garments. It's part of my life."

In the early 2000s, many companies began developing Velcro compression solutions for managing lymphedema. These Velcro solutions are called inelastic garments (not be confused with "elastic compression garments," or compression garments). They are made of a thicker neoprene fabric and are fastened with Velcro. They can deliver different levels of compression (20–30 mm Hg, 30–40 mm Hg, 40–50 mm Hg) to the limb, depending on how tight you pull the Velcro. They are often used as a transition-stage garment after bandaging, to get a further reduction in lymphedema volume before measuring for elastic compression garments.

If you can't tolerate bandaging, the Velcro garments can be used to reduce your lymphedema in the intensive phase of treatment (however, these may not work as well as bandages to reduce your lymph volume). Velcro compressions can be used instead of elastic compression in the maintenance phase in cases of pain, palliative care, arthritis, severe limb distention, and paralysis, and when it is simply not possible to get the elastic compression garments on.

Velcro compression garments do not require the same amount of strength to put on as elastic compression garments. They can be helpful if you are feeling especially weak or have severe arthritis or limited flexibility.

When additional pressure is needed, Velcro garments can be worn over your regular compression garments (this is known as layering compression garments). This can help you manage a flare-up of swelling or when flying in a plane — or other situations in which extra demands are placed on your lymphatic system.

You may find that your Velcro garments shift and slip during activity, especially when worn on the thigh area. Sometimes fluid collection can occur in the sections between the garment's straps. When you secure a Velcro strap, there is an overlap of fabric.

Velcro Foot and Calf Garments

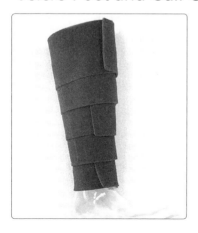
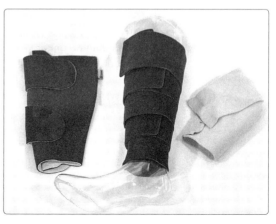

This double layer of fabric creates higher pressure and tends to push fluid into the area under the single layer of fabric. The fluid gets trapped and causes bulges in your limb. You may feel that it is hard to get the proper pressure gradient from the bottom to the top of the limb. (Special care should be taken to not pull some straps more than others; the pressure should feel the highest at the hand or foot so that a proper pressure gradient can be achieved.) To avoid these problems, nonslip underpadding and thick compression liners can be used.

➡ PRO TIP

A special anti-slip woven padding embedded with silicone or stretch foam can be used under Velcro garments to prevent them from slipping.

Layering Garments in Lymphedema

In some cases, it is helpful to put one compression garment over another. This layering produces an additional compression, but only an additional 70% of the top layer. For example, if your top garment is rated 20 to 30 mm Hg, adding it on top of your bottom layer contributes an additional 14 to 21 mm Hg pressure (70% of 20 to 30). Some clients might use a Velcro garment over their regular compression stocking; others might layer short-stretch bandages (the ones used in the intensive treatment phase of bandaging) on top of their compression stocking or sleeve to help control swelling when they are more active. This is especially helpful for ankle and hand swelling. Layering should be done only in consultation with your lymphedema therapist.

Nighttime Compression Garments

Typically, nighttime compression garments can be helpful for people with primary lymphedema. People with secondary lymphedema can benefit from using nighttime garments as well, but it depends on the severity of the lymphedema, pain levels and whether your lymphedema does not reduce when lying down. Nighttime compression garments have a lower pressure and do not fit as snugly as daytime compression. This lower pressure is needed because of the lower pressure of the vascular system when lying down. There are many options for nighttime compression garments.

Do you need nighttime compression? (Not everyone with arm or leg lymphedema will need to use this kind of self-care.) You will need nighttime compression if:

- Your lymphedema does not decrease during the night.
- You have dense fibrotic areas in your lymphedema.
- You have some other unique situation that may benefit from nighttime compression.

It is always best to consult with your lymphedema therapist to determine if this treatment option is appropriate for you.

LIVING WITH LYMPHEDEMA

"My morning routine is: I don't put my garments on in the morning; instead, I go straight to the pool. I keep my night wraps on until I am just about ready to leave the house. I have an accessible parking permit; the only time I use it is when I am at my pool without my stockings on."

Arm and Leg Garments for Nighttime Use

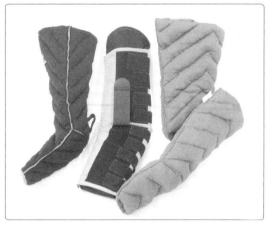

Nighttime compression options for the leg and arm.

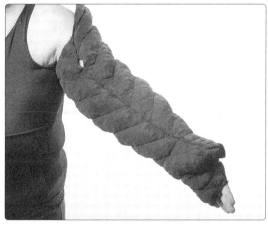

This option has channels full of foam chips, which help break up any existing dense tissue.

FAQ

Q. Are compression stockings or sleeves (either flat knit or circular knit) suitable for nighttime use?

A. No. Resting pressure in the vascular system decreases when you are lying down, so wearing a compression stocking or sleeve at nighttime could inadvertently restrict your blood circulation. You should sleep with nighttime garments, with bandages or with no compression at all.

Compression for Breast or Chest Wall

After breast cancer surgery and radiation, a significant number of people experience swelling or lymphedema of the breast or chest wall

After breast cancer surgery and radiation, a significant number of people experience swelling or lymphedema of the breast or chest wall. This swelling can cause pain, tightness, hardness or mobility issues, such as reduced shoulder mobility.

The chest wall can be a very difficult area to compress. Over-the-counter and custom-made vests are available (with or without sleeves); foam can be added to these to increase pressure in a congested area. The chest wall can also be compressed with long-stretch or short-stretch bandages cut to size by your lymphedema therapist. Foam padding can also be put underneath in areas where more pressure is needed.

Research Review: Compression for Chest Wall Lymphedema

A study conducted in 2016 with 37 women examined the use of a low-pressure compression corset to treat patients after mastectomy and lymph node removal. The aim of the study was to determine if a low-pressure corset could prevent the development of chest wall lymphedema. The low-pressure corset (18.98 mm Hg) was made of soft, flexible fabric, and its inner lining provided micro-massage (meaning that the corset rubs against your skin when you move, which acts similarly to MLD). Each corset included a side support and a prosthesis insert to exert more pressure. It had a high back and underarm openings that provided good pressure to the armpit and back areas.

Nineteen women received a compression corset 1 month after surgery, while the remaining 18 participants were placed in the control group (they did not use a corset). The women were measured at four different intervals and were followed for 7 months in total. Ultrasound was used to evaluate the thickness of the skin and the underlying layers of the chest wall.

In the final measurements, 7 months after surgery, the researchers saw significantly less thickness in the chest wall in the group that used corsets compared to the group that did not use them. (Some women also had radiation while enrolled in the study, and the researchers saw positive results in those women as well.) In the corset group, there was less swelling at 7 months and 58% of participants had less pain in the chest and shoulder girdle. In the group that did not use the corset, the researchers saw increased rates of swelling at 7 months and only 33% had less pain at 7 months.

The study found that 100% of all people in the control group developed lymphedema in the chest wall 7 months after surgery. The results suggest that compression corsets with 18.98 mm Hg pressure (called Class-1) could reduce pain and prevent chest lymphedema in patients with mastectomies following surgical lymph node removal. There are many compression vests and bras on the market, so speak to your lymphedema therapist or fitter to find one that has the proper fit for your body shape. These are made by the garment manufacturers that also make sleeves and stockings.

Compression for Genitals

There are several options available to help prevent and treat lymphedema of the genitals. You can use full-panty compression garments with or without custom-made foam inserts to increase the pressure in the genital area. Gray foam is another option, which can be put into pantyhose to help increase pressure in the areas that need it. Sanitary napkins, either one layer or two layers thick, are also an inexpensive and readily available option that you can use

> ### LIVING WITH LYMPHEDEMA
> *"I have to wear a bra, a vest and special underwear, and then I can function. If I don't wear them, I have to do extra manual lymphatic drainage, which takes too much time. I'd rather just put them on right after I get up."*

> *There are many compression vests and bras on the market, so speak to your lymphedema therapist or fitter to find one that has the proper fit for your body shape.*

between two pairs of underwear for vaginal or scrotal lymphedema. The thicker, cheaper pads provide more pressure and bulk than the expensive ones, which tend to be thinner.

Scrotal compression pouches like the Whitaker pouch can be used, or bike shorts can be worn to give extra support. When leg lymphedema accompanies genital lymphedema, care needs to be taken when compressing the legs so that lymphatic fluid does not pool in the genital area; proper genital compression needs to be achieved to prevent further pooling in the genitals.

Here is a list of additional recommendations to help treat genital lymphedema, supported in part by the research performed by Boris and colleagues in 1998:

- Bike shorts over bandages help hold bandages up and reduce genital swelling.
- A good athletic supporter, such as a jock strap, is good for scrotal or penile lymphedema.
- Combining compression with deep breathing exercises can reduce pubic and genital lymphedema. Deep breathing exercises open up the deep abdominal lymphatic pathways so that more lymphatic fluid can be cleared from the lower abdomen and genitals.
- Lying on your back with your feet elevated can also help.

Compression for Suprapubic Swelling

The suprapubic area is the area above the genitals, and lymphedema in this area can be treated with:

- Gray foam and channel foam
- Pantyhose compression with extra support in the suprapubic area
- Over-the-counter compression bike shorts worn over thigh-high stockings

It is important to consider your comfort level and your activity when adding extra support to the area above the genitals.

Compression for Head and Neck

Many different compression garment options exist for head and neck swelling. You can purchase over-the-counter and custom-made garments for many kinds of swelling in this area. Head and neck lymphedema needs to be compressed very carefully because of the arteries in the neck. People with head and neck lymphedema need to have sufficient blood flow through these arteries before compression can be considered. Speak to your head and neck surgeon prior to using compression for head and neck lymphedema to make sure it is safe for you to use.

In most cases, head and neck swelling tends to be worse at night, while sleeping; as a result, compression is used at night. Full-face masks with openings for the mouth, eyes and nostrils can be used if significant facial swelling is present. Chin straps can be used for swelling that is localized mostly to the area under the chin. Below are two examples of facial compression options.

Neck and Chin Compression

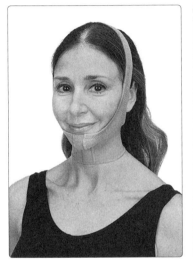 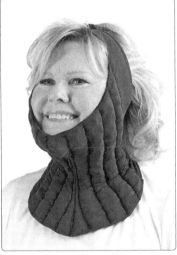

Various therapist-made solutions can be created easily for simple cases of swelling in the neck or under the chin as well. For example, short-stretch bandages can be cut to fit (and reused). A second option is to use stretch foam, which has the advantage of being easy to use and clean. Stretch foam is a good choice to use as a trial to see how your swelling will respond and to see if you can tolerate the compression. If this solution works, more expensive, long-term options can be purchased. Open-cell or gray foams can be added to either of these two options.

The Bottom Line

You and your lymphedema therapist need to work together to determine your individual compression needs, and the person measuring and fitting you for your garments needs to be properly trained. In order for your compression to be effective, you need to wear it long-term, and in order to do that, the garment needs to be comfortable and appropriate for you and your needs. There is no benefit to a beautiful compression garment that lies in your dresser unworn.

CHAPTER 7

Pneumatic Compression Pumps

While wrapping bandages around your lymphedema limb might seem like a very low-tech technique, pneumatic pumps are the ultimate in high tech. Pneumatic compression pumps are electronic devices that deliver pressure through a sleeve that inflates with air. To use one, you place your swollen arm or leg into the sleeve, turn on the device and wait while it inflates with air, applying pressure to the swollen limb. There are three types of pumps.

Single-Chamber Pumps

- There is only one chamber in the sleeve; it inflates entirely and deflates entirely.
- This kind of pump does not provide graduated compression.
- These models were the first pumps developed and are very rarely used.

Multi-Chamber Pumps

- The pumps can be programmed to deliver different amounts of pressure for as long as you need.
- The sleeve inflates upward from the foot or hand toward the hip or shoulder, and it deflates from the hip or shoulder to the foot or hand.

Multi-Chamber Pumps with Trunk or Central Chambers

- These pumps are similar to multi-chamber pumps; however, they are designed to first decongest the central zone (trunk) before moving to the swollen limb.

It might sound appealing to put your feet up or rest your arm on a comfy couch, watch some television and let a pump gently apply pressure to your limb while you relax, but it is not that straightforward. If you are considering the use of a pump as part of your lymphedema management plan, you will need to make an informed decision.

The general consensus in the lymphedema community is that pumps should not be used as a sole treatment option and should not be used as a replacement for complete decongestive therapy.

> **DID YOU KNOW?**
>
> The word "pneumatic" means "operated by air under pressure." In the case of pneumatic compression pumps, the air under pressure is within the sleeve.

> **LIVING WITH LYMPHEDEMA**
>
> *"For people with primary lymphedema, their lymphedema is different. Their body is used to pumps. When you have lymph nodes removed from surgery, like in secondary lymphedema, suddenly your body has to learn what to do."*

Furthermore, exercise, MLD or self-MLD and compression garments need to be used after treatment with a pneumatic compression pump. Some individuals who have primary lymphedema (an improperly formed lymphatic system) use pumps at night while sleeping and continue with compression stockings and self-MLD during the day.

When Pumps Can't Be Used

If you have one or more of the medical conditions listed here, you should not use pneumatic compression pumps.

- Acute inflammation of the skin (such as cellulitis or erysipelas)
- Cancer that has spread (metastatic) and has moved into the area with lymphedema
- Cardiac failure (uncontrolled or severe)
- Deep vein thrombosis (known or suspected)
- Edema at the root of the affected limb or truncal edema
- Ischemic vascular disease
- Non-pitting chronic lymphedema on a limb with a wound
- Peripheral neuropathy (severe)
- Pulmonary edema
- Pulmonary embolism
- Skin wounds (infected, undiagnosed or untreated)
- Thrombophlebitis

Caution is required for cases of:

- Extreme limb deformity (may impede the correct use of compression pumps)
- Fragile skin, skin grafts and skin conditions that may be aggravated by compression
- Limb pain or numbness
- Peripheral neuropathy

> **CAUTION**
>
> Generally speaking, patients with secondary lymphedema are advised not to use a pneumatic compression pump: the lymphatic system has been altered by surgery or radiation and this means that the uncontrolled movement of fluid to the top of the limb is not an effective way to clear lymphatic fluid (it may pool at the top of the limb). Manual lymphatic drainage achieves better results.

Research Review: Pneumatic Compression Pumps

The National Lymphedema Network (NLN) issued a position paper (a summary statement) in 2011 on their investigation into pumps. The paper reports that pumps should not be used without also doing complete decongestive therapy (CDT). There is concern that pumps remove excess water from the interstitial spaces (the spaces around the cells) but leave the protein behind. This results in a concentration of protein. Over time, water is drawn out of the blood vessels to dilute the protein and this increases the swelling in the tissues. This scenario (a higher protein concentration) is thought to cause the formation of fibrotic tissue, or fibrosis (thick scar tissue), thereby causing further damage to the flow of lymphatic fluid.

To investigate the hypothesis that a high protein concentration in the interstitial spaces leads to fibrotic tissue, a team of researchers from Brazil in 2001 examined the legs of subjects after treatment with a pump. They found that fluid accumulated at the top of the leg after the pump treatment. This fluid accumulation caused the development of a fibrotic ring at the top of the leg, which acted as a barrier to the flow of lymphatic fluid.

Another research team, this one from the United States in 1998, found that genital swelling was also seen in a large number of individuals after using a pump (compared to patients who underwent conventional CDT treatment). This is likely attributed to the uncontrolled forceful movement of lymphatic fluid into the genitals and abdominal area.

One concern that has yet to be investigated is whether the potential for cellulitis infections could increase if the proteins remain concentrated in the limb; studies have shown that bacteria can thrive in this protein-rich lymphatic fluid.

A second concern with pumps is that you have to be careful with how much pressure is applied to the skin: too high a pressure can damage the lymphatic vessels and further limit lymphatic flow. This was investigated by a couple of research teams, who found that a significantly higher pressure was delivered to the limb than was indicated on the control panel of some machines. It is very important that a physician or lymphedema therapist familiar with your lymphedema prescribes the settings for you and oversees the pump administration. It is always best to start pump treatment at a lower setting and then adjust as required.

STUDY #1

In 2014, a team of researchers from China conducted a systematic review of randomly controlled trials that compared the effectiveness of pumps versus CDT in reducing swelling in patients with breast-cancer-related lymphedema. The authors determined that there was no significant difference between CDT and pumps. They concluded that the trials failed to show that pumps were any better than traditional management strategies for lymphedema, such as bandaging and manual lymphatic drainage.

STUDY #2

A study published in 2001 from a team in Brazil examined the use of pumps to reduce leg lymphedema; the study also used lymphoscintigraphy (medical imaging for lymph nodes) to look at the lymphatic transport of proteins. The study involved 11 patients with leg lymphedema (stage 1 to 3, primary or secondary) who were between 25 and 75 years old. The individuals had suffered from lymphedema from as few as 1.5 years up to 29 years. Only one leg was treated with a pneumatic compression pump, whether or not participants had lymphedema in one or both legs.

Testing involved lymphoscintigraphy, a compression pump for 3 hours, and a second lymphoscintigraphy 48 hours later. The results revealed a reduction in the circumference of the leg — but only in the ankle and lower leg, not in the thigh. The authors hypothesized that the pump prevented lymph formation and moved the water out, but it likely did not remove the proteins from the leg, because the swelling returned.

STUDY #3

A study conducted in 1998 in the United States involved 128 people at risk of genital lymphedema due to their existing leg lymphedema. Seventy-five people did not use a pump for their leg lymphedema and 53 did use a pump. The results showed that 2 people (3%) out of the 75 who did not use a pump developed genital lymphedema, whereas 23 people (42%) of the 55 who used a pump developed genital lymphedema — and that genital lymphedema persisted after the pump was stopped. The incidence of lymphedema was not affected by the type of pump used, the pressure level used or the length of time the pump was used in a particular session.

The author's conclusion is that pumps used to treat leg lymphedema produce a high rate of genital lymphedema.

Ann's Clinical Experience

In my clinical practice, we do not recommend the use of pumps; the disadvantages of pump usage outweigh the advantages. Very few of my patients have used compression pumps to treat leg lymphedema; for those who have, I have sometimes seen genital or trunk swelling as a result. I have also seen patients who have developed neck, face or chest swelling from using pumps to treat arm lymphedema. I've even seen a few cases in which the use of a pump led to a fibrotic ring around the upper thigh area, which led to more blocked lymphatic pathways and a greater collection of lymphatic fluid.

The Bottom Line

Many people seek a "quick fix" solution for their lymphedema, but it is not recommended to use just a pump to manage your lymphedema. The use of pumps should be limited to a select number of cases of primary lymphedema — and only as an adjunct treatment when combined with CDT in the maintenance phase. The research continues on pump usage in lymphedema management, but some early studies show that thickened tissue and genital, head, neck or trunk swelling can occur. Use caution: not everyone with lymphedema will respond the same. Consult a lymphedema therapist or a physician knowledgeable about pump use before trying a pneumatic compression pump, and make sure the desired effect is achieved through prescribed settings and routine monitoring.

LIVING WITH LYMPHEDEMA

"I rented a pump; I used it for a week. I thought: unless someone gives me some guidance, I don't want to touch it. I don't want to make something worse."

CHAPTER 8

Exercise and Lymphedema

CAUTION

Many health conditions, such as heart conditions, can make it unsafe to exercise, so it is important to get medical clearance from your doctor before starting a new exercise program. Everyone is unique and will experience the effects of exercise in a different way, so begin any exercise program slowly and cautiously, monitoring for symptoms.

In the past, people with lymphedema were told to rest and limit exercise; however, there are newer research studies that support the safe, effective use of exercise for people with lymphedema or people at risk of lymphedema. Today, exercise is one of the four key elements that make up complete decongestive therapy (CDT), the gold-standard therapy for the treatment of lymphedema.

Exercise is essential for general health and well-being. There are many known benefits associated with regular exercise, such as improved strength, range of motion, endurance, immune function, health and body weight. In this chapter, we build on your understanding of the physiology of the lymphatic system, described in earlier chapters, to help you understand why exercise is such an important component of your lymphedema management.

Different exercises are usually recommended in the different phases of lymphedema treatment. In the intensive phase of treatment (while bandaged), remedial exercises are used. These kinds of exercises involve repetition with no weights, such as shoulder shrugs, elbow bends, hip flexes and ankle circles. Once the intensive phase has been completed, you don't need to restrict yourself to remedial exercises. In the maintenance phase, you may be able to return to some of the exercise routines and sports you enjoyed before your lymphedema developed.

Not everyone with lymphedema has had cancer; in fact, only about 15% of people with lymphedema had cancer first. But most of the research on lymphedema and exercise has been done with women after breast cancer. If you don't have breast-cancer-related lymphedema, you can still learn something about your own lymphedema from the research covered in this chapter, but you should also rely on the clinical experience of your lymphedema therapist. Your lymphedema therapist can help guide your decision about what and how much exercise you can safely participate in to receive maximum benefit.

Types of Exercise

The three main categories of exercise are:

1. Cardiovascular exercises (walking, hiking, running, swimming)
2. Strength exercises (weight lifting, resistance-band training)
3. Stretching exercises

Each category of exercise has its own list of benefits, but make sure to follow the guidelines outlined below so that lymphedema flare-ups can be limited or avoided.

Exercise during the Intensive Phase

When performing remedial exercises while bandaged, it is important to make sure you have good range of motion in your joints, you are achieving muscle contraction and your bandages do not limit your movement. Safety with exercise is important during the intensive phase, so do not perform any exercise you feel might not be appropriate for you. If you have concerns, speak to your lymphedema therapist.

In a clinical review by Galantino and Stout in 2013, 10 high-quality studies were pooled that looked at the effect of early versus delayed postoperative exercise following breast cancer surgery. Early exercise — performed in the first 3 days — was more effective than delayed exercise in the recovery of shoulder range of motion (achieving a full range of motion after surgery is extremely important because a loss of range of motion is a risk factor for developing lymphedema). No evidence was found to show an increased risk of lymphedema from exercise at any time after surgery for breast cancer.

Since most of the research is done on breast cancer patients, we don't know if the same results will apply to surgeries on other areas of the body, such as the neck, abdominal area or leg. Your postoperative plan of care is dependent on many factors, such as type of surgery, use of drains, and complications that may develop; follow the protocol of exercise given by your surgeon.

Exercising during the Maintenance Phase

Nearly all forms of exercise can be modified so that they can be performed safely and effectively by people with lymphedema during the maintenance phase, but make sure to check with your lymphedema therapist before starting a new exercise. If you have been diagnosed with lymphedema, exercise should be performed

➡ **PRO TIP**

Here are some tips to keep you exercising:

- Start a program you know you can continue.
- Choose an exercise you enjoy doing.
- Find a buddy or partner to help you stay motivated and to encourage you.
- Plan exercise into your daily routine.

while wearing your compression garments. Start with a very short period of time, such as 5 to 10 minutes, and progress slowly. Of course, past exercise and general fitness levels will play a big role in what the start of your exercise program looks like.

Start with 2 sets of 10 to 15 repetitions of an exercise and progress every 2 to 3 weeks provided all is going well (no heaviness in your limb, no aches, no pins and needles, no increase in your swelling). Typically, you should exercise 2 to 3 times per week, with 2 days of rest in between — but everyone is different. Design your exercise routine with your lymphedema therapist.

If you are beginning a weight-lifting program, perform the exercise first with no weights for 1 to 2 weeks. If, following this period, you are symptom-free, add weights at the lowest amount and increase weight gradually.

Muscle and Joint Pumps

Professors Michael and Ethel Földi were pioneers in lymphedema treatment and were the first to define muscle and joint pumps.

The muscle pump occurs when the contraction of muscle increases lymphatic fluid movement. To stimulate the muscle pump, you must perform active exercises (rather than passive ones). Compression garments and bandages further improve the efficiency of lymph flow while exercising, called a positive working pressure. Weak muscles result in less muscle pumping and less fluid movement; because of this, it's important to include strengthening exercises as part of your exercise routine.

The joint pump can be activated with active or passive movements. Its full effect is achieved if you have a full range of motion in your joint (a reduced range of motion limits the effectiveness and results in less lymph clearance).

To maximize the benefits of both the muscle pump and the joint pump, work with your lymphedema therapist to create a plan that treats any existing mobility issues and improves your range of motion and muscle weakness. Implement this plan as part of your complete decongestive therapy (CDT) to achieve the best results.

Decongestive Exercises

Decongestive exercises are ones that remove excess fluid (decongest) while wearing bandages or compression garments. Professors Michael and Ethel Földi recommend following this protocol for exercise:

1. Perform self-manual lymphatic drainage before beginning your exercise session.

2. Do 20 to 30 repetitions of warm-up exercises for large joints, such as the hip or shoulder.

3. Begin your exercise sequence as follows:

- For upper body, begin with your shoulder (proximal end) and move to your fingers (distal end). Contract the muscle when you **inhale**.

- For lower body, begin with your hip (proximal end) and move to your toes (distal end). Contract the muscle when you **exhale**.

4. Perform one or two stretching exercises per muscle. Be sure to hold the stretch for 20 to 30 seconds.

Below and on the pages that follow, you'll find a list of decongestive exercises that you can use as part of your lymphedema management and overall healthy living plan. Bring this book with you to your appointment with your lymphedema therapist so they can coach you on which exercises and techniques are best for your unique situation, including your balance, strength and prior level of activity. If you have poor balance, hold on to a firm surface, such as a railing or countertop, to perform these exercises.

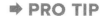

➡ PRO TIP

Perform deep-breathing exercises throughout the day to relax your diaphragm and help with lymphatic fluid movement.

Ann's Clinical Experience

I use decongestive exercises in my clinical practice to help people during the intensive phase. We do standing exercises because they are functional exercises (exercises that help you have more stamina for regular daily activities). These can be incorporated into your day at home or work. The lying positions can be done when you wake up in the morning or before you go to bed.

LEG EXERCISES
Exercise 1: Hip Adductors

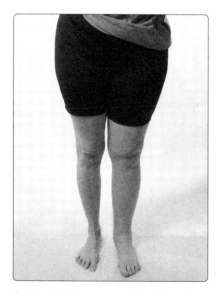

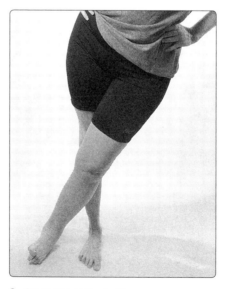

Alternative method: Lie flat on your back and put a small pillow between your thighs so that your legs are hip width apart; squeeze the pillow for a count of 3 seconds and then relax.

1. Stand with your feet shoulder width apart.

2. Cross your affected leg over your unaffected leg as far as you can while you breathe out. Return to the starting position as you breathe in.

Exercise 2: Hip Abductors

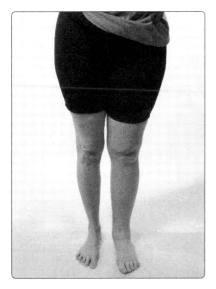 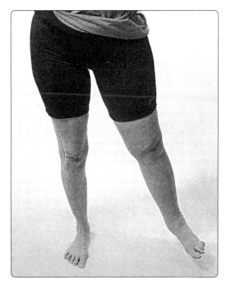

Alternative position: Lie flat on your back and move your leg straight out to your side with your toes facing the ceiling.

1. Stand with your feet shoulder width apart.

2. Lift your leg out to the side, with your knee straight and your toes pointing straight ahead, as you breathe out. Return to the starting position as you breathe in.

Exercise 3: Hip Flexors

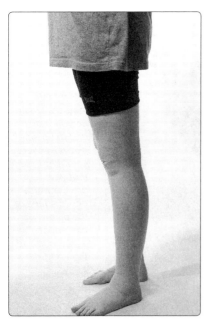 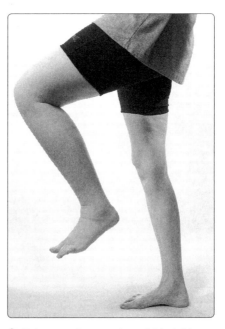

Alternative position: Lie flat on your back and slide your foot toward your buttocks, raising your knee to the ceiling.

1. Start with your feet shoulder width apart.

2. Raise your knee up to waist height (toward 90 degrees) as you breathe out. Return your leg to the starting position as you breathe in.

Exercise 4: Knee Flexion

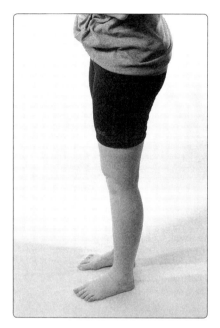 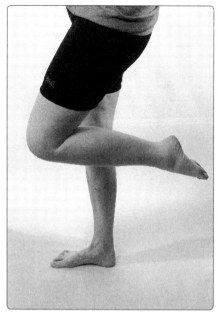

Alternative position: Lie on your stomach and raise your foot toward your buttocks by bending your knee.

1. Stand with your feet shoulder width apart.

2. Bring your foot up toward your buttocks by bending your knee as you breathe out. Lower your foot to the ground as you breathe in.

Exercise 5: Ankle Range of Motion

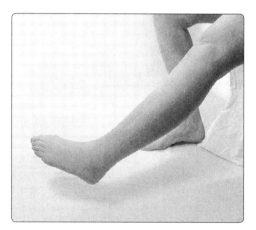 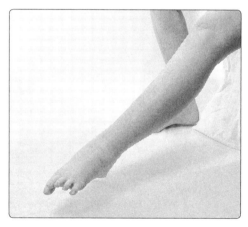

1. Sitting with your foot raised off the ground, rotate your foot inward and make small circles.

2. Roll your foot outward.

Alternative position: Lie flat on your back and make circles with your ankles, one at a time.

Exercise 6: Toe Crunches

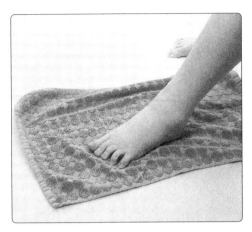 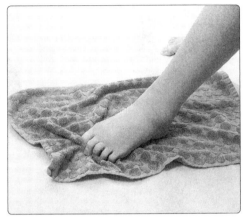

1. In a sitting position, place your foot on a thin towel.

2. Wrinkle up the towel by crunching your toes together, as if you are trying to pick up the towel with your toes. Then spread the towel out with your toes, back to the starting position.

Exercise 7: Heel Raises

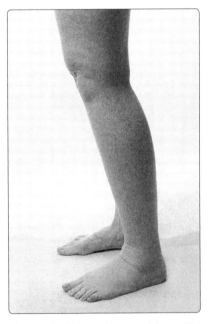 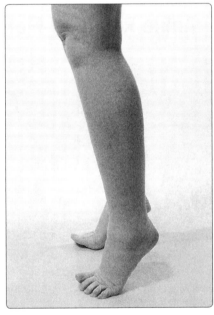

Alternative position: Lie flat on your back and point your toes, alternating feet, as if to press on the gas pedal of the car.

1. Stand with your feet shoulder width apart.

2. Rise up onto your toes as you breathe out, and return to your starting position as you breathe in.

Exercise 8: Step-Ups

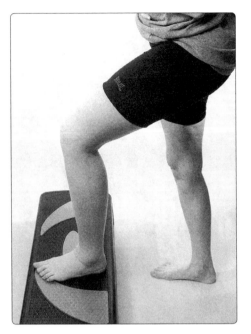

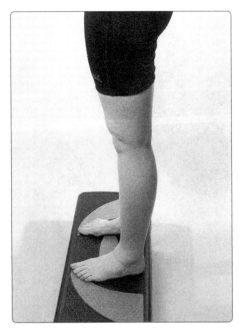

1. Stand with your feet shoulder width apart. Place your foot on the first riser of your step (if you have leg lymphedema, start with your lymphedema leg).

2. Bring your other foot up to the step while you breathe out. Then return back to the start position as you breathe in.

> ➡ **PRO TIP**
>
> While many lymphedema therapists are physical therapists (physiotherapists) and therefore have a strong background in exercise sciences, as you may recall from "Who is qualified to help me manage my lymphedema?" on page 28, people from many different professions, such as a massage therapist or an occupational therapist, can become certified as a lymphedema therapist. Talk to your therapist about their comfort level in prescribing exercise and don't be afraid to ask for a referral if this is not something they are comfortable assessing and prescribing.

Exercise 9: Chair Squats (Sit to Stand)

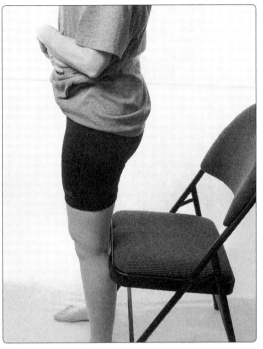

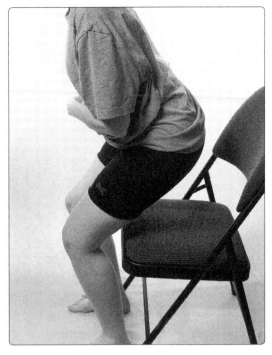

1. Stand in front of a chair with your feet shoulder width apart. If you have poor leg muscle strength or balance, a chair with armrests can be used for support.

2. Bend at your knees and hips while aiming your buttocks to the back of the chair.

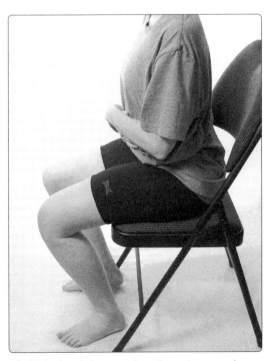

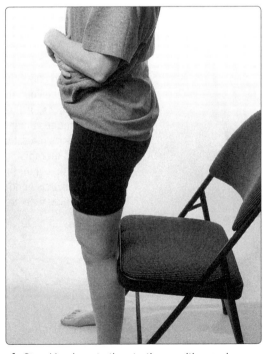

3. Sit in the chair as you breathe out.

4. Stand back up to the starting position and breathe in.

ARM EXERCISES
Exercise 1: Shrugs

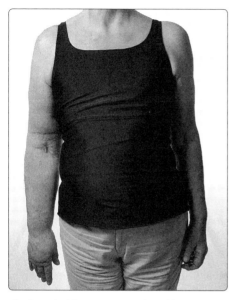 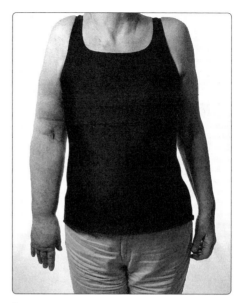

1. Stand with your arms relaxed by your side.

2. Shrug your shoulders up as if trying to bring your shoulders to your ears as you breathe in. Return to the starting position as you breathe out.

Exercise 2: Shoulder Abduction (Side Raises)

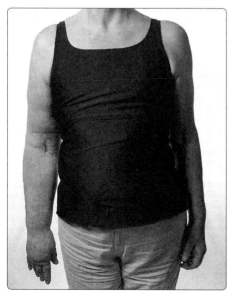 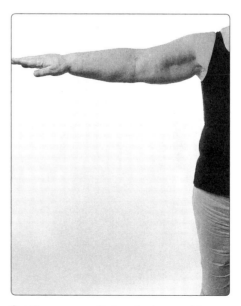

1. Stand with your arms relaxed by your side.

2. Lift your arm with lymphedema out to the side, up to shoulder height, as you breathe in. Lower your arm back to the starting position as you breathe out.

Exercise 3: Shoulder Flexion (Front Raises)

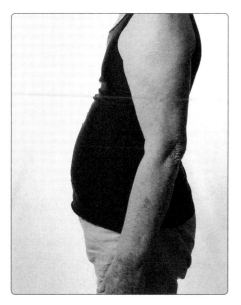

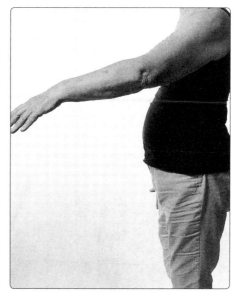

1. Stand with your arms relaxed by your side.

2. Keeping your arm straight, raise your arm with lymphedema in front of you, up to shoulder height, as you breathe in. Lower your arm back to the starting position as you breathe out.

Exercise 4: Elbow Flexion

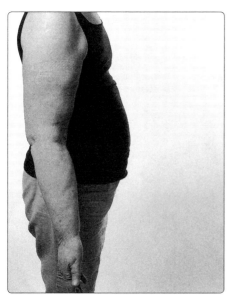

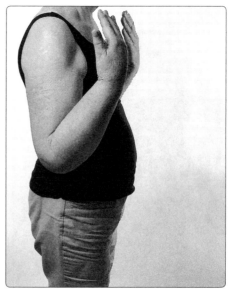

1. Stand with your arms relaxed by your side, palms facing forward.

2. Bend at the elbows and bring your hands as close to your shoulders as you can as you breathe in. Return to the starting position as you breathe out.

Exercise 5: Wrist Flexion

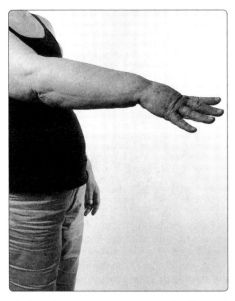 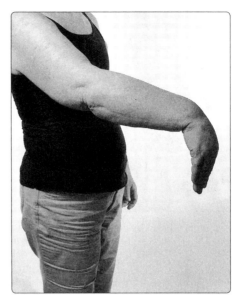

1. Stand with your arm extended in front of you, palm facing down.

2. Bend at the wrist to point your fingers to the ground as you breathe in. Return to the starting position as you breathe out.

Exercise 6: Grip/Make a Fist

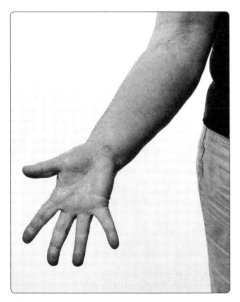 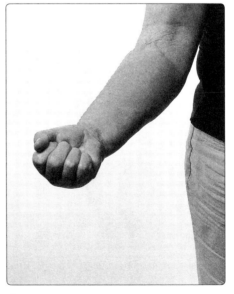

1. Start with your arm relaxed, fingers splayed open.

2. Make a fist with your hand as you breathe in. Open your hand as you breathe out.

Alternative exercise: Squeeze and release a small, malleable ball in your hand.

Exercise 7: Bilateral Shoulder Abduction

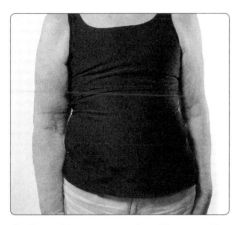

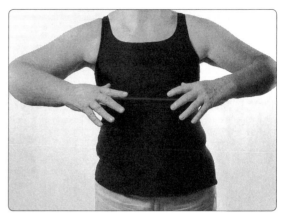

1. Start with your arms relaxed by your side.

2. Bend your elbows and bring your hands up to in front of your ribcage with your fingers reaching toward each other as you breathe in (the movement should come from the shoulders). Return to the starting position as you breathe out.

Exercise 8: Lateral Torso Stretch

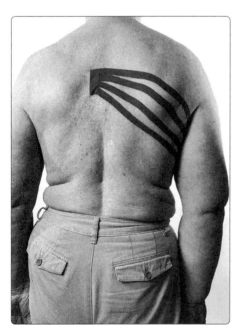

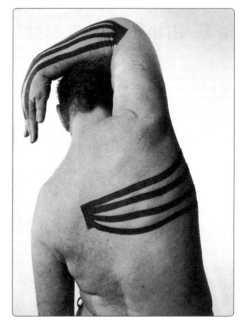

1. Stand with your arms relaxed by your side.

2. Reach your hand over your head and down toward your opposite shoulder as you breathe in. You should feel a slight stretch along the side of your body. Return to the starting position as you breathe out.

Exercises Studied for Lymphedema

Researchers have studied numerous exercises to determine their effectiveness in improving lymphatic flow. Below is a selection of the exercises that clients ask about most often: pool exercises, yoga, Nordic pole walking and strength training. Exercise is an important part of CDT, but this is the part that is often skipped. This sample of evidence should help reassure you that exercise is safe and hopefully get you motivated!

Research Review: Exercise and Lymphedema

Baumann and colleagues in 2018 did a systematic review of the research on exercise for breast-cancer-related lymphedema. A systematic review involves finding all the research published on a topic and pooling the results to determine the best recommendations. This review looked at 11 randomized trials totaling 458 women. The exercises included aqua therapy, swimming, resistance training, yoga, aerobics and gravity-resistance exercises. None of the studies showed any adverse effects on lymphedema. Four studies showed a reduction in swelling and six studies showed decreased fat, increased muscle, increased strength, increased arm range of motion, weight loss and improved quality of life. This is good news for people with breast-cancer-related lymphedema: it means you don't need to fear exercise and can look forward to some measurable benefits. Likely the same is true for lymphedema due to other causes, too. Here is a representative sample of research done on those four exercises.

Pool Exercises

When you get into the pool, the water acts as compression for your lymphedema. The deeper you go in the water, the more pressure you'll feel — which is beneficial. Because of the natural compression, you don't need compression garments or bandaging. As a bonus, you get to enjoy a break from wearing them.

If you're interested in giving water exercise a try, contact your local fitness or community center and see what types of pool programs they offer. Start off slowly with only a short session of 20 to 30 minutes and increase your duration as your fitness level improves. If you experience any unusual symptoms, such as heaviness, aching or pins and needles, discontinue the activity and speak to your lymphedema therapist.

Here is one study to highlight the safety and benefits of pool exercise for lymphedema.

DID YOU KNOW?

The tissue in the area of the lymphedema has less blood supply and more fat deposits.

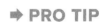

➡ PRO TIP

The pool water temperature should be between 68°F and 86°F (20°C and 30°C).

*"When I'm in the
pool, I can exercise
without the heavy-duty
stockings. I can do
squats and lunges in
the pool, but I can't do
those on land with my
leg lymphedema."*

*"The pool is the best!
You don't need to
be wrapped."*

Research Review: Pool Exercises

Johansson and colleagues in 2013 investigated the effects of water-based exercises on arm lymphedema and shoulder range of motion in breast cancer survivors. They randomly assigned 15 women to a group that performed pool exercises and 14 women to a control group (routine activity). The water-based exercise group was given six specific exercises that needed to be performed in the water each time and could be repeated if time allowed. They were also instructed to swim or stretch but told that each session should last 30 minutes and should be performed 3 times a week.

The researchers found no significant effect on the lymphedema of the water-based exercise group, with the exception of two participants, who had a limb volume reduction between 25% and 32%. Researchers did find that the water-based exercise group had a significant improvement in arm range of motion even when the exercise was performed up to 10 years after completing their cancer treatment. None of the women in the water-based exercise group had a worsening of lymphedema; this supports the idea that water-based exercises can safely be performed by women with arm lymphedema after breast cancer treatment.

Yoga

Yoga is a form of exercise that incorporates deep breathing, stretching, range-of-motion movements and strengthening poses. There are many different types of yoga, such as hatha and Bikram. Yoga's benefits include a reduction in stress, increased joint range of motion, improved strength and flexibility. Hatha is a gentle type of yoga that is slow and easier for people with lymphedema. If you have leg lymphedema, you may find chair yoga easier to perform; standing poses and sitting on a floor mat may make yoga difficult.

You might think there are a lot of studies to show the benefits of yoga for lymphedema. Surprisingly, there are only about a dozen studies — and they have similar results: yoga doesn't make lymphedema worse and it produces a temporary improvement. Here is a sample of one of the yoga studies.

What to Avoid

Lymphedema patients should avoid these yoga situations:

- Hot yoga (the room temperature can cause a flare-up of lymphedema)
- Poses that require a lot of strength
- Prolonged time in one pose
- Downward dog
- Head and shoulder stands

Research Review: Yoga

Loudon and colleagues in Australia in 2014 conducted a study of 23 people with Stage 1 arm lymphedema. The participants were divided into two groups. The first group of 15 people attended a group Satyananda yoga class (breathing, physical postures, meditation and relaxation) once a week for 90 minutes and were given a yoga DVD to watch daily. The second group of 13 people served as the control group and were told they were on the waiting list and just to continue their usual exercise, whatever that was. People in the yoga group were given a choice of wearing a compression sleeve for the yoga sessions.

The yoga lasted for 8 weeks, after which no reduction of lymphedema was seen (but also no increase). There was, however, a decrease in scarring (fibrosis) in the upper arm in the yoga group compared to the control group. Four weeks after stopping the yoga, that difference in scarring was no longer evident. On the down side, there was an increase in lymphedema a month after stopping yoga.

This study shows that fibrosis could be initially reduced with yoga, but a month after stopping yoga, there was no longer an improvement. There was also increased swelling in the arm with lymphedema. According to this study, it appears that doing yoga is not a problem for lymphedema, but stopping it might be. Keep this in mind if you are planning changes to your exercise routine.

> **LIVING WITH LYMPHEDEMA**
>
> *"Exercise is like a pump. The more you move, the more you pump your lymphatic fluid."*
>
> *"I did yoga for 10 to 15 years, but in yoga, you hold your poses for too long, so I don't do that anymore. Now I do water walking and tai chi."*

Beneficial Yoga Poses

There are some Internet resources available that demonstrate beneficial yoga poses for lymphedema (such as www.lymphedemablog.com). Here are some poses you can try at home:

- Elevated legs up the wall: lie on your back, feet on the wall
- Half-standing forward bends: bend forward at the hips and stretch out your arms parallel to the floor
- Simple hand movements: raise your hands over your head and breathe deeply
- Cat–cow pose: while on your hands and knees, arch the back upward, then downward

Nordic Pole Walking

Nordic pole walking has been growing in popularity in Europe for the past 20 years. It has been slow to gain popularity in North America, but it has many benefits, including:

- The six-step protocol is easy to learn and affordable, as you only need to buy the poles (no gym membership required).
- It reduces the impact on your lower extremities because some of the force goes through the poles while walking.
- This activity activates 90% of your body's muscles.
- You can burn a lot of calories with this exercise; it has been shown to burn more calories than walking, running or cycling.
- It uses the muscle pump, helping to stimulate increased lymphatic fluid clearance.

Research Review: Nordic Pole Walking

Nordic pole walking has been investigated for its safety and benefit for breast-cancer-related lymphedema. Jonsson and colleagues in 2014 conducted a study to investigate the effects of Nordic pole walking on arm lymphedema and cardiovascular fitness in women after breast cancer. Twenty-three women completed three to five sessions (each session was 30 to 60 minutes) of Nordic pole walking per week for 8 weeks (24 to 40 sessions in total). The researchers found that arm lymphedema was significantly reduced at the completion of the study. They also found that there was an improvement in overall cardiovascular fitness.

Proven Health Benefits of Nordic Pole Walking

- Decreased resting heart rate
- Decreased blood pressure
- Increased exercise ability
- Improved oxygen uptake by the lungs
- Increased quality of life
- Weight loss

In addition to the benefits listed above, Nordic pole walking has been shown to increase upper body strength. If you don't see results early on, don't give up — you may need up to 24 sessions to see improvements. In fact, in 2016, researchers in Italy determined there was no benefit with just 10 sessions of Nordic pole walking and suggested that you need time to learn the proper technique.

It has been suggested that the reason North Americans are slower to take up the sport of Nordic pole walking is that you may feel you look silly doing it. But Nordic pole walking has been shown to have a more positive effect on arm lymphedema than walking alone, so perhaps it's time to give it a try.

Strengthening Exercises

Breast cancer patients have long been advised to limit weight training as a form of exercise. However, these restrictions often remain in place only until 3 months after surgery or radiation; for special cases, the restriction may remain in place longer. The immediate postoperative limit is to restrict lifting to no more than 10 pounds (4.5 kg).

It is best to clarify with your surgeon or lymphedema therapist regarding what type of restrictions you have following each of your medical procedures and to know how long any restrictions last.

Advancing weight training in a slow and progressive way can be a safe and effective way to increase muscle mass and improve lymphedema. If you are new to exercise, start off with a lymphedema therapist to set up a program based on your individual needs.

Research Review: Strengthening Exercises

When it comes to lymphedema and strength training (also called weight lifting), the goal is to gain all the benefits of weight training without any negative effects on your lymphedema. Much research has been done in this area — most but not all of it in the breast cancer population. Here are three studies: one on breast cancer, one showing the benefits for prevention and one for leg lymphedema.

WEIGHT TRAINING AND BREAST CANCER

Zhang and colleagues from Philadelphia in 2017 wanted to determine the effects of weight lifting on lymphedema. A total of 141 women with arm lymphedema after breast cancer were used in the year-long study — 71 were in the weight-lifting group and 70 were in the control group. The researchers took baseline measurements of their arm lymphedema as well as fat, muscle and bone density measurements.

The study involved 13 weeks of 90-minute supervised weight-lifting sessions twice a week. The exercises included total body workouts (arms, legs and cardio) of 3 sets of 10 repetitions each. After 13 weeks, the women were given YMCA memberships to continue the exercises on their own. On the weight-lifting machines, they increased weights by the lowest increment possible — and only after two sessions with no change in symptoms. They wore their

DID YOU KNOW?

As lymphedema progresses, the swelling is transformed into scar tissue (fibrotic tissue) and fat.

DID YOU KNOW?

A program of controlled exercise with weight lifting may increase your muscle mass and your ability to do more activities with your lymphedema arm, thereby protecting the arm from injury during the common activities of daily living, such as cleaning, yard work and grocery shopping.

compression garments during exercise. After 1 year of weight-lifting exercises, lean muscle mass and bone mineral density increased and body fat decreased. The biggest increases in lean mass were seen in the women with less severe lymphedema. Despite all these benefits, there was no change in lymphedema.

These results are similar to other studies of exercise after breast cancer, which showed that — although about 10% of women did experience an increase in lymphedema (which was no different than the usual-activity control group) — the majority of participants had stable lymphedema with weight training.

WEIGHT TRAINING AS PREVENTION

A second year-long study, by Schmitz and colleagues, performed at the University of Pennsylvania School of Medicine in 2010, studied the risk of lymphedema development with exercise in patients after breast cancer treatment. The women's treatments had ended 1 to 5 years earlier and they had at least two lymph nodes removed. Seventy-two women did 13 weeks of twice-weekly 90-minute supervised group sessions of progressive weight lifting called PAL (physical activity and lymphedema). They were then given a 1-year membership at a local fitness center to continue an independent exercise program. Another 75 women served as the control group and did not exercise.

After 1 year, 11% (8 of 72) in the weight-lifting group developed lymphedema in the at-risk arm — as did 17% (13 of 75) of the women in the control group. Of the women who had five or more nodes removed, 22% (11 of the 49) of the control group and 7% (3 of the 45) of the weight-lifting group developed lymphedema. This study highlights that, while a small number of women developed lymphedema, the lymphedema was less in the exercise group compared to the control group. The study showed that a program of slowly progressing weight training did not result in any more lymphedema than no exercise, and this should reassure you that exercise is safe and may even be protective when you are at risk of lymphedema.

WEIGHT TRAINING AND LEG LYMPHEDEMA

A small clinical trial done to assess the safety of performing weight-lifting exercises in people with leg lymphedema was done by Katz and colleagues at the University of Pennsylvania in 2010. Ten people with leg lymphedema following cancer treatment participated in the study. The 5-month study involved 2 months of supervised group exercises, followed by 3 months of independent exercises at a local fitness center. Participants completed a full-body strengthening program, consisting of 90-minute sessions twice a week; each session included two or three sets of 10 repetitions for each exercise. On the weight-lifting machines, participants were allowed to increase weights by the lowest possible increment every two sessions so long as they suffered no symptoms of worsening lymphedema. After the study, those participants who completed the study showed very little change in their lymphedema but did experience an improvement in strength, walking speed and single-leg balance.

The Bottom Line

Exercise is an essential component to any healthy lifestyle. The benefits of exercise in general are very well known and well researched. However, the ideal exercise type and quantity to best assist with lymphedema still need to be fleshed out. It would seem from the studies available that the benefits of exercise outweigh the risks. Although the most commonly researched exercises were highlighted in this chapter, there are many other types of exercises. If you want to go square dancing, play water polo or go dragon-boat racing, go for it; don't limit your interests based on the limited research. Discuss any exercise you're interested in pursuing with your lymphedema therapist, and enjoy!

DID YOU KNOW?

People with lower leg lymphedema tend to move more slowly than healthy adults of similar age, likely because larger limbs are harder to move and they slow people down.

LIVING WITH LYMPHEDEMA

"It has to be personalized — when you do it, how you do it, how it fits into your life."

Lymphatic Taping

Lymphatic taping is a technique in which special medical tape is applied to the skin to direct the flow of lymphatic fluid. It is an emerging new option for the treatment of lymphedema and can be used in conjunction with bandaging and compression garments.

Taping was invented by a Japanese chiropractor and inventor named Dr. Kenzo Kase more than 30 years ago. He used taping to treat athletic injuries and to help with swelling. He hypothesized that applying the tape with a stretch of 5% to 15% could lift the skin, increase the space between the middle layer of skin (the dermis) and the collagen layer beneath the skin (the fascia), and decrease the pooling of lymphatic fluid by increasing lymphatic flow.

The tape was developed to be the thickness and weight of human skin so that it could mimic the skin's properties. It can move fluid from a congested area into a lymph node basin or another uncongested area of the body. It also has a massaging effect on the skin during physical activity and muscle contraction. In clinical practices, clients report less congestion, less heaviness and less pain in the area of congestion.

There are several advantages to taping, including:

- It is more comfortable (than compression garments) in hot weather.
- Taping can be used in certain conditions where compression cannot (for example, when fine motor skills or sterile conditions are required).
- It can be used on areas of the body that are hard to compress (for example, the abdomen, chest, head or neck).
- It can be used in situations where compression cannot be used (for example, for nerve injuries or numbness).

DID YOU KNOW?

If you have numbness, compression bandaging and garments aren't always safe. You need to be able to feel if your compression is too tight. If it's too tight, you could develop a wound (skin ulcer). Taping, on the other hand, can be used safely with numbness.

Not Just Any Tape

If you've ever watched the Olympics or another major sporting event, you've probably seen athletes wearing black or brightly colored tape directly on their skin. That is the same tape that is now being used to treat people with lymphedema. It goes by several names: kinesiology tape, kinesio tape, K-tape, physio tape, medical tape, sport tape, sport kinesiology tape and athletic tape.

The tape is 100% cotton and latex-free, and it has a medical-grade acrylic adhesive backing that is body-heat activated. It is both hypoallergenic and water resistant. During the manufacturing process, the tape is applied to its paper backing with a 10% stretch. When it is not on the paper backing, it can stretch another 50% to 70% in length (the tape can stretch only lengthwise). This stretch can be used to relax or stimulate muscle function.

As Dr. Kenzo Kase's tape (Kinesio Tape) has gained popularity in treating sports injuries, so, too, has the variety of brands on the market increased — such as Leukotape K, RockTape, SpiderTech, Kindmax and TheraBand kinesiology tape. Many brands can be purchased from medical equipment stores, pharmacies and online suppliers, and different brands vary by the amount of stretch, the type of adhesive and the quality. It is best to try a few types if the first one doesn't agree with your skin or doesn't stick well.

> **➡ PRO TIP**
>
> Most lymphatic taping is done without applying additional stretch (more than what the tape already has on the paper).

A Word of Caution

Lymphatic taping is not recommended for your lymphedema if you have one of the following conditions:

- Acute congestive heart failure
- Acute kidney disease
- Chronic renal failure
- Liver disease
- Skin treated with radiation (unless deemed appropriate)
- Unstable blood pressure
- Untreated blood clot (deep vein thrombosis)

Using tape in one of these conditions could inadvertently move fluid into an already struggling heart, kidney or liver (causing fluid overload); it can also move clots and damage irradiated skin.

If you have other medical conditions as well as lymphedema, please speak with your lymphedema therapist to determine if this treatment is safe for you and which taping application is the best for your particular lymphedema. It is always best to consult with your medical team or lymphedema therapist before starting a new treatment.

Research Review: Lymphatic Taping

There aren't a lot of high-quality randomized controlled trials on taping for lymphedema, and the studies tend to have a small number of subjects. Much of its use is based on clinical experience. This is an area that requires further study to support its use. The results in many studies vary — often because of low sample size, a varying length of treatment time (often too short), a varying length of follow-up (often too short), and inconsistencies in standardizing treatment protocols.

STUDY #1

In 2016, Martins and colleagues looked at the safety and tolerability of taping in 24 patients with arm lymphedema. Since none of the subjects had skin lesions, they were all able to have taping. Tape was applied on the full arm, chest and back. Although there wasn't a measurable improvement in their lymphedema, the condition didn't get worse and the majority of participants were pleased with its use for treatment and reported no change in social life or activities of daily living. On the negative side, 4% of the participants experienced skin peeling and redness, and 75% reported that the tape detached at the ends.

STUDY #2

In 2009, Tsai and colleagues studied 42 people living in Taiwan who had one arm with moderate to severe lymphedema for more than 3 months as a result of breast cancer treatment. The study participants were divided into two groups. The first group of participants was bandaged for their lymphedema and the second group was taped. Both groups also received 5 days a week of manual lymphatic drainage (MLD), lymphatic pump treatment and exercise.

The bandage group lost 1.1 ounces (33 mL) more volume than the taping group. It should be noted that the bandaging group kept their bandages on for only 7 to 8 hours per day — compared to the 23 hours per day that is usually recommended — so it is likely that a higher reduction in swelling would have been seen in this group if they had kept their bandages on longer.

In the end, the authors reported that taping was preferred over bandaging by the participants (likely because of the hot climate), and that taping did produce some volume reduction and reduced the density and hardness in the lymphedema. However, bandaging produced the better reduction in lymphedema.

	BANDAGE GROUP	TAPE GROUP
Reduced tightness	✔	✔
Reduced soreness	✔	
Reduced discomfort	✔	
Reduced fullness	✔	✔
Reduced pain		✔
Reduced hardness		✔
Reduced tingling		✔
Volume reduction	2.8 oz (84 mL)	1.7 oz (51 mL)

STUDY #3

In a 2014 Turkish study, Pekyavas's research team compared the results of three different treatment types, manual lymphatic drainage (MLD) plus: (1) bandaging; (2) bandaging *and* taping; or (3) taping. Included in this study were 45 people with moderate to severe lymphedema 6 to 8 years after surgery for breast cancer. All of the participants performed exercise and received 10 sessions of the specific treatments assigned to their group.

FOLLOW-UP	MLD + BANDAGING	MLD + BANDAGING + TAPING	MLD + TAPING
After 10 sessions			
Decreased volume	✔	✔	✔
Decreased pain		✔	✔
At 1 month			
Increased activities in daily living	✔	✔	✔
Decreased volume		✔	

There was no significant difference between all three groups in terms of pain, ability to perform daily activities, discomfort, heaviness, stiffness, numbness and quality of life — all experienced some improvements in these areas. But the group that received all three treatments (MLD, bandaging and taping) showed volume reductions that lasted the longest.

The researchers hypothesized that the reason for this was the dual effect of the lymphatic tape (which channeled the lymph fluid away) and the bandaging (which pumped the fluid away from the area) in addition to the MLD. The significant pain decrease in

the two groups that received taping was thought to be the result
of the lymphatic tape lifting the skin, which creates ridges or waves
that enlarge the area of the surface skin and free the nerve endings.
The study was limited to a small number of people per group and
participants had only 2 weeks of treatment. A longer study with
more participants may reveal different findings.

STUDY #4

In 2016, Taradaj's research team from Poland wanted to determine
the influence of taping on the volume of lymphedema and manual
dexterity in the arms of women after breast cancer treatment.
They wanted to determine if taping could replace bandaging. In
their evaluation, they assessed limb size, grip strength and range of
motion after 4 weeks of treatment. All three groups received manual
lymphatic drainage and lymphatic pump treatment; each group
was assigned one additional treatment: real taping, placebo taping
(it looked like real lymphedema tape, but wasn't) or bandaging.

	TAPING GROUP (22 PATIENTS)	PLACEBO TAPING GROUP (23 PATIENTS)	BANDAGING GROUP (25 PATIENTS)
Reduction in arm volume	22%	24%	45%
Range of motion	Slight increase	Slight increase	Largest increase
Strength	Slight increase	Slight increase	Largest increase

The authors found that lymphatic taping was not effective
at reducing limb volume in the subjects with Stage 2 and Stage 3
lymphedema. On the positive side, though, the range of motion in the
lymphedema arm increased in all groups. Bandaging also provided
improvements in grip strength, quality of life and limb use for
activities of daily living.

Getting Started

Many YouTube videos, DVDs and books can be found on lymphatic
taping techniques, but please use these resources with caution. It
is always best to consult a lymphedema therapist to make sure the
treatment is safe for you and your situation. A full physiotherapy
assessment of your current medical condition, past medical history
and your history of lymphedema is needed to determine if it's safe
for you.

Taping should not be your only form of treatment, because there
is not enough evidence to suggest that taping can replace complete
decongestive therapy, which is still considered the gold standard
of treatment. Taping can be used in addition to manual lymphatic

drainage and compression therapy (bandaging or garments), and it is best to use it in areas that are hard to treat with compression bandaging or garments, such as the abdomen, chest wall, torso, head and neck. Your therapist should explain everything you need to know about taping: why the tape is being used on a particular area of your body, where the placement of the tape should be, and if stretching of the tape is needed. It is important to know how and when to remove the tape. This is a time when your therapist can give you advice and pointers and ensure the correct placement of the tape. Once you understand your taping prescription, you can do your own taping at home. (It is advisable that at a follow-up visit with your lymphedema therapist, you and your caregiver demonstrate how you've been applying the tape, to make sure no adjustments are needed.)

It is worth noting that it's good to take a day off from taping; this allows the skin to breathe and allows for proper bathing so that all the residue from the adhesive can be removed. Over time, irritation or allergic reactions can develop. If this occurs, stop taping and follow up with your lymphedema therapist. It's possible that a different lymphatic pathway could be used for your taping.

Anchors and Tentacles

It is important to understand the direction in which lymph fluid will flow within the lymphatic system, so that the tape can be effective and can safely move the fluid away from the congested area. The end of the tape that the fluid will drain toward is called the anchor. Although we think of an anchor as something that keeps a ship from drifting, this anchor is pulling fluid toward it. The pieces of tape that draw the fluid out of a congested area and draw it toward the anchor are called the tentacles — a term created for the purpose of this book.

What to Know before You Tape

- Taping should not be used on very dry skin because the tape will stick too much and will remove some skin.
- Do not put the tape right over active malignant tumors.
- Do not put tape on thin skin (such as on people over 70 years old and people taking steroids or blood thinners; the skin can peel when the tape is removed).
- It is wise to test a small 1-inch (2.5 cm) area of skin to make sure that the skin won't peel when the tape is removed and that you are not allergic to the adhesive.
- See also "A Word of Caution" on page 115 for conditions that are not conducive for taping.

CAUTION

The instructions in the pages that follow are not inclusive of all the taping techniques used by lymphedema therapists. These should be used only in consultation with your therapist, who has determined — by assessment — which ones are best for you. Bring this book to your assessment and review which taping technique is right for you. Your therapist may add to, modify or delete some of the taping methods. These general steps do not replace a certified lymphedema therapy program or certification and should not be used by untrained or uncertified health-care workers to treat lymphedema patients.

Step-by-Step Guide to Taping

Before Getting Started

- Make sure the skin is clean, dry and free of lotions and oils.
- Ensure that the skin is cleared of hair. If you have a small amount of hair, the tape can be applied over it. If you have a significant amount of hair, it will need to be removed (with an electric razor) to make sure the tape adheres to the skin. Too much hair in the area also results in significant pain when the tape is removed.
- Make sure the skin where the tape will go has no wounds, open areas, rashes, blisters or peeling.

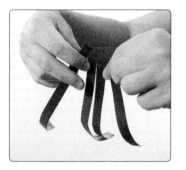

1. Cut the tape to the desired length, then cut the tentacles (if necessary), before applying to the skin.

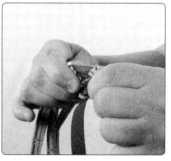

2 Identify where the anchor should be placed. Remove the tape from its paper backing in the anchor area by simply grasping the anchor and pulling. This will tear the paper backing, which you can peel off to reveal the adhesive.

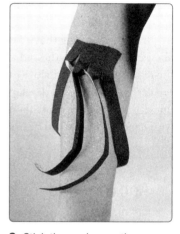

3. Stick the anchor on the area you want the fluid to drain to (for example, for hand lymphedema, place the anchor on the forearm).

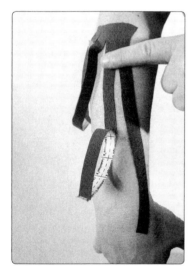

4. Position the body part you are trying to drain in a stretched position (for example, if you are draining your hand, straighten your arm by your side and make a fist with your fingers). Pull the paper backing from the tape along each of the tentacles, one at a time, and press them flat on the skin. There is no need to stretch the tape.

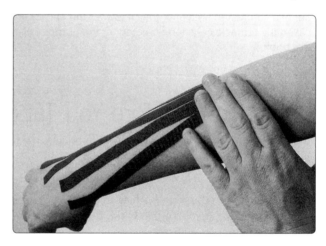

5. Rub the tape for about 30 seconds to 1 minute, through its entire length, to activate the adhesive.

Taping Tips

- Do not let the tape get wet for at least 1 hour after application; this will give the tape a chance to set against the skin.
- Do not wear compression garments in the area for at least 1 hour after application, to prevent the tape from rolling or curling at the ends.
- The tape can stay on the affected area for 3 to 5 days. It should be removed immediately if your skin becomes irritated, itchy or red, or if a rash develops.
- You can shower or swim with the tape on; simply pat the tape dry with a towel when you're done. Although it is waterproof, the surface does tend to feel a bit moist after prolonged exposure to water. It takes only a few minutes to dry.
- Do not blow-dry the tape; the heat will increase its adhesiveness and make it very hard to remove (if not impossible) without peeling off the top layer of skin.

Anchor and Tentacle Placement

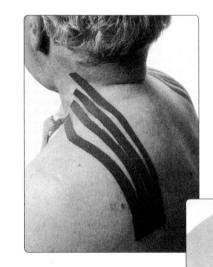

Head and Neck Swelling ⮞

The anchor is placed in the middle of the shoulder blade and the tentacles are extended upward to the side of the neck where the congestion begins.

Chest Swelling ⮞

This technique is used to help clear breast and chest wall swelling. The anchor is placed on the opposite side of the spine and the tentacles extend to the side of the chest where the swelling is. (This technique is used only when lymph nodes have been removed from one armpit, not both.)

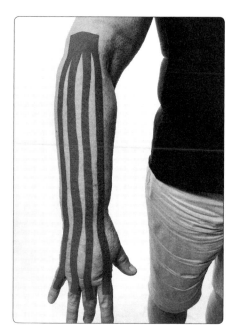

Swelling on the Back of the Hand

The anchor is placed on the outside of the elbow and the tentacles extend to the ends of the fingers. If finger swelling is also present, you can extend the tentacles down the finger.

Swelling on the Top of the Foot and Ankle

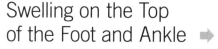

The anchor is placed behind the knee and the tentacles extend to behind the ankle, with two on each side, and ending on the top of the foot.

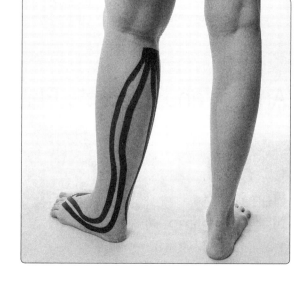

Upper Arm and Hand Swelling

The anchor is placed behind the shoulder and the tentacles extend around the front of the arm toward the inner elbow. The second anchor is placed on the forearm (as seen in Swelling on the Back of the Hand) and the tentacles extend to the back of the hand.

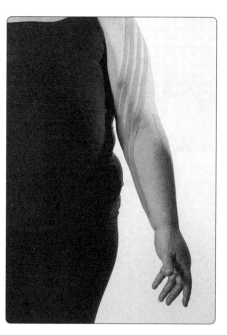

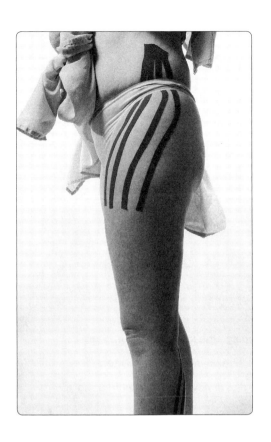

← Swelling in the Leg or Thigh for Someone Using Thigh- or Knee-High Compression

The anchor is placed below the ribs and the tentacles extend down the outside of the leg to the top of the stocking.

Swelling in the Foot → and Calf Area

The anchor is placed on the mid-thigh on the back of the leg and the tentacles extend down to behind the ankle and to the top of the foot.

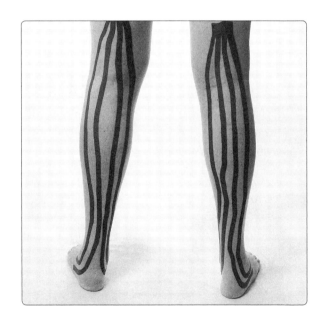

HOW TO: Remove Lymphatic Tape

1. When it's time to remove the tape, use your index finger to gently peel one of the corners (see arrow) and then use the palm of your hand to brush the rest of the tape off with a stroking motion, just like brushing something off your arm.

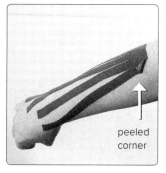
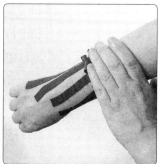
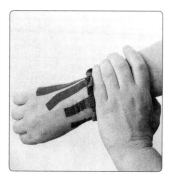

peeled corner

2. Do not pull the tape off like a Band-Aid, as it will damage the top layer of skin.

3. It is not advisable to remove the tape in the shower, as skin damage is likely to occur.

4. The tape should be removed when it is completely dry; removing it just before a shower means you can wash off any leftover adhesive on your skin.

5. If the tape is hard to remove, rub olive oil or baby oil on the tape for several minutes to saturate the entire length of it. This will help loosen the tape from the skin.

LIVING WITH LYMPHEDEMA

"K-tape doesn't work very well for me if I am wearing compression stockings. It detaches and rolls up my leg."

The Bottom Line

Taping can be used as a safe strategy for managing lymphedema and you should discuss how it can be added to your individualized lymphedema treatment plan with your lymphedema therapist. Its effectiveness is not fully known, as the research studies show mixed results and often involve too few people to prove their benefit. If you have no medical issues preventing you from using tape, consider doing a trial with your therapist to determine if it is a good tool for you in managing your lymphedema.

PART 3
Nutrition for Lymphedema

CHAPTER 10

Body Weight and Lymphedema

Of all the nutrition topics, weight loss has the most research to support its role in reducing lymphedema. It's important that you understand how your weight can impact your lymphedema, so this chapter gives you added insights that will empower you with the knowledge to take your health into your own hands. You'll better understand that what and how much you eat can have a positive impact on your lymphedema, and you'll also find recommendations for how to move your body weight in a healthy direction.

Research Review: Body Weight
STUDY #1

In October 2007, a study was conducted in London, England, to investigate whether dietitian-guided weight loss would add benefit to the treatment of breast-cancer-related lymphedema.

Participants were required to have a body mass index (BMI) greater than or equal to 25 kg/m^2 and their lymphedema arm had to be more than 15% larger than their unaffected arm. Twenty-one women with breast-cancer-related lymphedema were randomly divided into two groups. The first group (the control group) received a booklet on general healthy eating. The second group received dietary advice from a registered dietitian and were seen twice during the 12-week study to make sure they were still following the diet.

The women who received guided instruction on a weight loss diet were advised how to eliminate 1,000 calories from their usual intake, and the diets were all in the range of 1,000 to 1,200 calories per day. No exercise or activity guidelines were provided.

Results

After 12 weeks, the results were tallied. The women in the weight-loss group lost an average of 7.3 pounds plus or minus 5.7 pounds (3.3 kg plus or minus 2.6 kg), whereas the control group did not lose weight. These results were certainly expected.

To see if this had any impact on lymphedema, the researchers compared excess arm volume. The group that received the individualized low-calorie weight loss diet instruction (and lost the weight) experienced a significant reduction in excess arm volume — 12 ounces (350 mL). The women in the control group did not.

> ➡ **PRO TIP**
>
> Excess arm volume is the difference in arm volume between the arm with lymphedema and the healthy arm.

STUDY #2

In a May 2007 study by the same researchers in London, England, 51 women with breast-cancer-related lymphedema were divided into one of three groups:

1. Control group (no change in diet or exercise)
2. Low-fat group (low-fat diet, but not low-calorie; designed to maintain weight)
3. Weight loss group (low-calorie diet designed to lose weight)

The goal was to compare two different diets and see whether a low-fat diet or a low-calorie diet would be better for reducing lymphedema.

Results

After 24 weeks, there were significant differences in the reduction of body weight, BMI (body mass index) and percentage of body fat between the control group (no diet) and the other two groups. There was also a slightly greater reduction in excess arm volume in the two diet groups. Results showed that the biggest difference in lymphedema didn't depend on the diet type, though; it did, however, depend on whether the women lost weight or not.

Interestingly, weight loss did not occur as predicted. Nine women (60%) in the control group lost weight, and 13 women (76%) in the low-fat group lost weight — even though the study was designed so that neither of those groups would lose weight. It's possible that the idea of being in a research study made them more conscientious about what they were eating. Eighteen women (95%) in the weight loss group lost weight, which is what was predicted.

In this study, there was a significant difference in the reduction of lymphedema based on weight loss — and it did not matter which of the three diets was used. The bottom line? Weight loss can reduce lymphedema.

FAQ

Q. Why does obesity contribute to lymphedema?

A. While the answer to this is not yet known for certain, some ideas put forth by research from the October 2007 British study opposite suggest:

- Increased body fat may reduce the efficiency of the muscles responsible for pumping the lymphatic vessels.
- The deeper levels of lymphatics are buried below a thicker layer of fat.
- Excess weight may limit the effectiveness of compression bandaging or garments.

SUMMARY OF BODY WEIGHT AND LYMPHEDEMA

You have the power to make improvements in your lymphedema by making changes to your body weight.

While there are only two clinical trials that have been conducted to specifically investigate the effect of weight loss on existing lymphedema, there are a further 11 studies that show that being overweight (BMI of 25 or more) or obese (BMI of 30 or more) is a risk factor for the development of lymphedema (see References, page 264).

Most of these studies involved participants who had had cancer treatment, and the goal was to determine why some people develop lymphedema after cancer and others don't. The nutrition risk factor that showed up consistently was that those who were more overweight after their treatment had a greater likelihood of developing lymphedema. Read more about this in Chapter 2: Lymphedema Risk Reduction.

Although you may not have the opportunity to lose weight before surgery (any surgery that would remove or damage lymph nodes) or before radiation treatment, losing weight after the procedure can help reduce your risk before lymphedema develops.

You have the power to make improvements in your lymphedema by making changes to your body weight. In addition to all the great strategies discussed in Part 2 of this book, nutrition offers you even more tools to help you manage your lymphedema.

Top 10 Tips to Help You Lose Weight

There are many strategies that you can incorporate into your routine to help you lose weight in a healthy way. Here are 10 proven weight loss tips.

1. Pay Attention to Your Feelings of Hunger and Fullness

The continuum in the illustration opposite represents the different levels of hunger and fullness that you might experience during your day. A good weight loss strategy is to avoid the ends of this continuum and stick to the middle. This means that you should be feeling hungry-peckish when you have your first meal of the day and you should eat until you are satisfied. Then, 3 to 4 hours later, you may find yourself feeling peckish again and should eat either a snack or lunch until you are satisfied. You continue this pattern throughout your day until your evening meal. It takes time for your brain to register these changes in your feelings, so eat slowly and tune in.

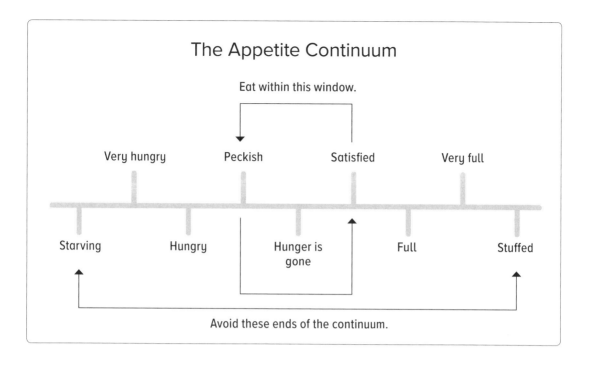

The Appetite Continuum

Eat within this window.

Very hungry — Peckish — Satisfied — Very full

Starving — Hungry — Hunger is gone — Full — Stuffed

Avoid these ends of the continuum.

2. Avoid Overeating and Feeling Famished

This is much easier to accomplish if you avoid letting yourself get too hungry. When you are at this stage, you have zero impulse control. Picture this: You have left work or home and you are rushing to get somewhere; you are very hungry and likely a bit dehydrated — as well as feeling tired and drained. You need to stop for gas and when you pay at the checkout, you notice that chocolate bars are on sale — two for $1.50. Without thinking much, you grab two. Before you even get back to your car, you have opened the wrapper and taken your first big bite. That is an example of zero impulse control.

The Layers of the Lymphatic System

Carrying extra body fat increases the distance between the layers of the lymphatic system, and the deeper layers become buried under a larger fat layer. This distorts the vessels so that there are kinks in the vessels, slowing down lymphatic flow.

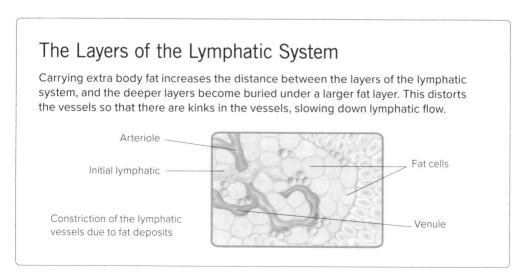

Arteriole

Initial lymphatic

Fat cells

Constriction of the lymphatic vessels due to fat deposits

Venule

When you live in an environment where junk food is available every place you go, eating healthily can be very difficult. How do you protect yourself from overeating? Avoid the feeling of extreme hunger. The best way to do this is to eat every 3 to 4 hours, choose meals that include fiber-rich foods and proteins, and drink plenty of fluids.

3. Balance Meals and Snacks

Your body is designed to maintain balance (or homeostasis) in your blood sugar levels. When you cut back on what you eat, it's important to maintain the balance in your food choices. You want to avoid low-blood-sugar symptoms such as cravings, crankiness, an inability to concentrate and a lack of energy. Balancing your meals and snacks with carbohydrates, healthy fats and proteins can minimize these symptoms.

When you cut back on what you eat, it's important to maintain the balance in your food choices.

What Are Carbohydrates?

Carbohydrates are starches and sugars. Grains (bread, rice, corn), sugars, milk, fruits and root vegetables are all important sources of carbohydrates. Your body breaks down carbohydrates into their smaller, single-sugar form for absorption; most commonly this is glucose (also called dextrose), but it can also be fructose or galactose. Carbohydrates are a main source of fuel for metabolism. Think of metabolism like the body's engine.

LIVING WITH LYMPHEDEMA

"As my lymphedema has progressed, drinking alcohol triggers a flare-up for me."

What Are Healthy Fats?

Healthy fats include vegetable-based fats such as vegetable oils, nuts and avocados. Read more about this in Chapter 12.

DID YOU KNOW?

Lipedema can be a metabolic, inflammatory or hormonal disorder. It is characterized by fat deposits that accumulate throughout the body, mainly affecting both legs and/or both upper arms; it has a characteristic "shelf" appearance on the upper buttocks and a "cuff" on the ankles and/or wrists. It affects mainly women and its onset is usually around times of hormone changes. Symptoms include tenderness, pain and swelling (it is sometimes called "painful fat syndrome"). Like lymphedema, lipedema is a chronic condition, but it can also be treated with complete decongestive therapy. Lipedema, like obesity, can also be a cause of lymphedema because it increases the distance between the layers of lymphatic vessels, which become distorted by fat deposits.

What Are Proteins?

Proteins are the building blocks of cells, including the cells in muscles and organs. With digestion, food proteins are broken down into amino acids, which are then small enough to be absorbed through the intestines and transported into the blood. The amino acids are then transported to the cells and rebuilt back into proteins. These proteins can be used as energy for muscle, cartilage, skin, blood, immune cells and other important cells. Dietary protein can be found in meat, fish, eggs, dairy, legumes and nuts. Smaller amounts are also found in grains.

Each meal should contain whole grains, protein and vegetables in at least equal proportion. If not equal, vegetables should take up the largest portion of your plate.

Balance Meals with Carbohydrates (Whole Grains), Proteins and Vegetables

Like many things in life, balance is key when it comes to the three main food groups in your meals. Each meal should contain whole grains, protein and vegetables in at least equal proportion. If not equal, vegetables should take up the largest portion of your plate.

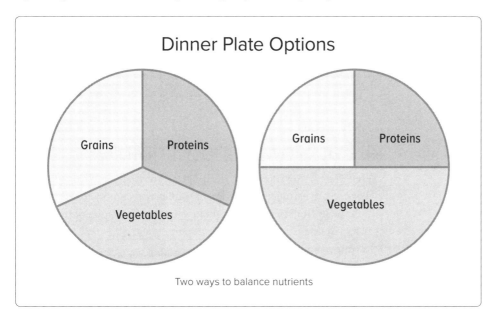

Dinner Plate Options

Grains / Proteins / Vegetables

Grains / Proteins / Vegetables

Two ways to balance nutrients

Balance Snacks by Including Carbohydrates, Proteins and Healthy Fats

Roasted chickpeas, edamame beans, unsweetened yogurt and tuna with whole-grain crackers are all snack ideas that contain carbohydrate, protein and healthy fat. When you eat a snack that contains carbohydrate, protein and healthy fat, your blood sugar level rises more slowly, which provides a more sustained energy level and appetite control. Including low-carbohydrate vegetables in your carbohydrate- and protein-rich snack is also great.

Benefits of Balance

- **Provides more stable blood sugar:** Some people experience increased hunger or cravings after a carbohydrate-heavy meal (think midafternoon sweet cravings and low energy levels). To avoid this, make sure to always eat a balanced meal and snack. This works because proteins and fats are slower to leave the stomach, and when carbohydrates are eaten at the same time as proteins and fats, the rise in blood sugar following carbohydrate digestion is slower, too.

- **Holds your appetite longer:** A balanced meal or snack will leave you feeling satisfied for longer after a meal. This helps protect you from going too far toward the starving end of the appetite continuum.

- **Keeps and builds muscle:** If you don't eat enough protein, your body can break down your own muscles to use for protein. You don't want this. You want to maintain your muscle mass and hopefully build new muscle; doing so is a major component of your body's ability to respond to acute and chronic illness, and it helps to repair injuries and produce immune responses. Although you need to exercise to build muscle, combining carbohydrates and protein after a workout is the best combination for muscle building. The carbohydrates will raise your blood sugar and insulin levels, and then the insulin will help the protein get into your muscles where it's needed.

4. Eat Slowly and Mindfully

What does eating mindfully mean? It means that you pay attention to what you are eating and you don't mindlessly pick up whatever food might be in front of you throughout your day. Examples of mindless eating would be:

- Eating out of boredom or some emotion you are feeling
- Eating when you aren't hungry
- Eating because you don't want to waste the food on the table
- Eating to finish the food on your plate because that was the way you were raised, even though you already satisfied your hunger several bites before
- Eating while doing other things (such as watching TV or surfing the Internet) to the point that you barely register the eating experience

Why should you eat slowly and mindfully? You may find this hard to believe, but your body knows exactly how many calories it needs. Eating mindfully involves really enjoying your meal and appreciating everything that you are sensing. This includes the appearance of the food, the aromas, the flavors, the way each bite feels in your mouth. When you do this, you become aware of the moment

FAQ

Q. I've heard the ketogenic diet can help with my lymphedema; is this true?

A. The ketogenic diet is a high-fat, moderate-protein and low-carbohydrate diet. This diet has been used for decades in children and adults with epilepsy and there is renewed interest in this diet in the weight loss, diabetes and cancer communities. No research to date has been published on the use of a ketogenic diet for lymphedema. The ketogenic diet does show benefit for weight loss, and therefore you could hypothesize that the diet could help you improve your lymphedema through weight loss. Although this hypothesis is reasonable, it is not a slam dunk. Without evidence for the ketogenic diet in lymphedema, it is not known what the outcome would be, and it would be interesting to know how the high level of long-chain fatty acids in the ketogenic diet might impact the lymphedema (see Chapter 11: Lymphatics and the Digestion of Dietary Fats for more information).

There is a video presentation on the Lymphatic Education and Research Network website (www.lymphaticnetwork.org) that describes a small 3-month intervention with 18 people, six of whom followed a ketogenic diet. Those participants lost both weight and limb volume. However, details about the comparison diet were not outlined; if the comparison diet was a typical North American diet, this would be a high-salt, inflammatory, weight-promoting diet, so a lot of diets would show good results against that. Also, if the main benefit for lymphedema is from the weight loss, it's not clear if a ketogenic diet would be helpful if you have lymphedema but a normal or only slightly above-normal body weight. It would be prudent to work with a registered dietitian who is knowledgeable about the ketogenic diet if this is something you want to try. In this way, you could make sure you are following the diet properly, your lab values can be monitored, you can deal with diet side effects and, finally, you are monitoring your lymphedema to know if you are achieving results.

at which your enjoyment starts to decrease — this is your body telling you that you've had enough. If you aren't paying attention to your eating, if you're focused more on how much food is on your plate, or if you eat too fast, you miss the signal. Eating slowly is important because it takes time for your brain to register that you've had enough.

DID YOU KNOW?

In English, we say "I'm hungry" and "I'm full." In French, they say "J'ai faim" and "Je n'ai pas faim" ("I have hunger" and "I don't have hunger"). Try to eat until you no longer have hunger, and don't focus on eating until you are full.

5. Make Your Home, Car, Commute and Office Safe

A common comment people share when they struggle with weight loss is "I can't lose weight because I don't have enough willpower." What an uncomfortable way to try to lose weight! Having to use your willpower to keep you from eating can be incredibly draining and makes focusing on other tasks difficult. To counter this, keep your home, car, commute and office as safe as possible. What does this mean? Here are some examples of changes some of our clients have made in their daily routines to keep themselves safe:

→ PRO TIP

It really helps if you can get others on your side in your journey to lose weight, especially the people you live with. When you're at home, you want to be able to relax and feel safe; if tempting food is around, especially in plain sight, then coming home after a bad day can turn into a really bad night for your weight loss goal.

- Alice no longer walks by the desk of her co-worker who always has a candy dish on display.
- Patricia now drives a different route to her mother's home every weekend, so that she doesn't have to pass the donut shop on the way.
- Beth asked her husband to buy only ketchup-flavored chips, as that is the one flavor she doesn't like.
- Imani no longer goes into the boardroom at work if she knows there was a meeting and the leftovers are up for grabs.
- Shawn takes a different route to his commuter train at the end of the day so that he doesn't walk past the ice cream shop.
- Nadia spoke to her husband and kids about what foods they can bring home and which cupboard they can be stored in.
- Sharon buys only a single serving of a treat. For example, if she wants ice cream, she buys one ice cream bar rather than a carton of ice cream or a box of bars, even though it's not as economical.
- Nathan and his wife agreed that, when they entertain, they will send their guests home with the treats that they brought and won't keep those tempting foods in the house.
- Iris stopped keeping treats for her grandkids in the kitchen, knowing that she will eat them between visits; instead, she gets stickers and other little gifts for them and serves them a special healthy snack.
- Jack volunteers to be the designated driver after sports practice so he won't be tempted to drink beer after the game.

Don't make weight loss any more difficult than it has to be by putting yourself in the way of temptation. Keep healthy snacks in the glove compartment, in your desk at work and in a bowl on the kitchen counter at home. The easier it is to grab, the more likely you will be to eat healthy options. Carry a BPA-free water bottle in your purse or backpack.

6. Focus on What You Should Eat and Not What You Shouldn't

Whatever type of improved health results you're aiming for — weight loss, lower cholesterol, lower blood pressure, reduced lymphedema — you can make it easier on yourself by thinking about all the food you *should* be eating (not the food you *shouldn't* be eating). This is a powerful psychological tool because it helps you maintain a positive relationship with food. Here is a list of foods that you can include in your diet every week:

You can make it easier on yourself by thinking about all the food you should *be eating (not the food you shouldn't* be eating).

- Whole grains (such as rolled oats, wheat berries, quinoa, barley, buckwheat and amaranth)
- Legumes (such as lentils, beans, peas, chickpeas and tofu)
- Vegetables (eat all of them, at every lunch and every dinner; aim for one-third to half of your plate)
- Fruit (eat all of them; aim for 2 to 3 spread throughout your day)
- Healthy oils (such as organic canola oil, flaxseed oil, extra virgin olive oil, avocados and nuts; read more about oils in the next chapter)
- Fish (especially salmon, sardines, herring, mackerel and rainbow trout)
- Herbs and spices (eat all of them; try to include an herb or spice at every meal)
- Plain probiotic yogurt, kefir and other fermented foods (such as tempeh, sauerkraut and kimchi)
- Grass-fed meats cooked at lower temperatures and without charring

When you focus on incorporating these healthy foods into your diet, you will find that your plate is full of healthy foods and you'll gradually squeeze out the unhealthy foods. This definitely requires support from the rest of the people in your household, so take time to talk to them about how they can support you.

7. Track Your Intake

One tool that many people find helpful is a food diary. This tool will help you become more aware of what you are eating. If you are reluctant to write down a particular food, you are less likely to eat it. There are lots of apps that can not only serve as a food diary but can also add up your calories, as well as the macro- and micronutrients, such as carbohydrate, protein, fat, sodium, vitamins and minerals.

Jean's Clinical Experience

As a registered dietitian, I see the progress that clients make when they work with me to lose weight, as well as the problem-solving skills they develop when they encounter challenges or setbacks. I recommend enlisting some professional help. As one of my successful clients recently told me, "If I could have done it myself, I would have!"

See if there is a registered dietitian in your area whom you can meet with face-to-face — or someone you can work with virtually. Working with clients on the phone allows me to offer support, ideas and accountability and it's super convenient for my clients.

You can search for a dietitian at one of these organizations:

- In the United States: Eat Right Academy of Nutrition and Dietetics, www.eatright.org
- In Canada: Dietitians of Canada, www.dietitians.ca
- In the United Kingdom.: Association of UK Dietitians, www.bda.uk.com

Many employee-benefit plans cover part or all of the cost of a registered dietitian; check with your insurance plan to confirm. If it's not covered, speak with your HR department and let them know this is of interest to you and advocate for future coverage. In the meantime, make the investment in your health and don't put off beginning your sessions.

8. Move More

To reduce cancer risk, current guidelines for the general public recommend exercise 225 minutes a week. (People with lymphedema should progress slowly to this guideline and monitor for flare-ups.) This works out to about 30 minutes every day or 45 minutes five days a week. Set a goal for yourself to go for a walk or do some other activity every day, and build up to 30 minutes for each session. If you are already doing this and not getting the results you want, increase the duration, the frequency or the intensity of this activity. For example, if you want to increase the duration, do 40 or 50 minutes of exercise instead of 30 minutes one day of the week, then build up to more days per week. If you want to increase the frequency, go for two walks instead of one a week, then build up to more days per week. Increasing intensity involves working harder in a fixed amount of time. There are a variety of methods for increasing intensity; here are some ideas to get you started:

- Add intervals to your walk. Once you have warmed up, do a 1-minute power walk. Slow down for 3 minutes to recover, then repeat another 1-minute power walk. Repeat this pattern throughout your walk.
- Use walking poles while you walk. The increase in arm movement increases your calorie burn.

- Add lunges to your walking routine. Do lunges every 10 minutes. Start with 10 repetitions in each set, then increase every week.

- Wear a backpack with a weight.

- Find a walking route that includes stairs or a hill climb.

9. Resistance Train to Increase Muscle Mass and Metabolism

Adding resistance training to your routine can do a lot to encourage weight loss. This is especially effective for postmenopausal women. We start to lose muscle mass starting at age 20, but these losses accelerate with menopause. Rebuilding muscle helps keep your metabolism going strong, and it helps prevent falls and bone loss. Check out Chapter 8: Exercise and Lymphedema for examples of exercises you can do.

⇒ PRO TIP

If you are constrained by time, you can still get the results you need. Many of these techniques to increase intensity can be used for running, cycling, rowing and other activities. Check with your lymphedema therapist for an appropriate personalized exercise plan that is best for you and your lymphedema management.

FAQ

Q. I've tried to lose weight before and I always gained it back; why would this time be any different?

A. For many people, the difficulty with a weight loss program is not losing the weight; it's keeping it off. For her book entitled *Thin for Life: 10 Keys to Success from People Who Have Lost Weight and Kept It Off*, author Anne Fletcher interviewed people who had lost at least 20 pounds (9 kg) and kept it off for at least 3 years, to determine if there were commonalties among these successful weight losers. The average weight loss was 63 pounds (29 kg), and most had kept it off for at least 5 years.

Common strategies were found to be a low-calorie, low-fat diet; regular (sometimes daily) weighing or keeping food records; a high level of physical activity (mostly walking); eating breakfast; not buying things they didn't want to eat; stress management and social support. The good news is that these successful weight losers reported that weight maintenance became easier over time, and if they were able to maintain their new weight for 2 to 5 years, it greatly enhanced their chances of long-term success. These successful weight losers advised readers to maintain behavior changes, make a commitment to a sustained lifestyle and take the view that this is a lifelong process, and, most importantly, believe that they can achieve weight loss.

10. Start with the Easiest Change First

Chances are you've already thought of some changes that you could make to help yourself lose weight. Some of those changes you may be dreading, but some may seem really easy. Start with the easy changes first. It's a good idea to roll out the changes one at a time. Read through the list again and think about how easy or difficult each of these would be for you. Make a list and put them in order from easiest to most difficult; you may need to modify this list as you implement changes, but this will give you a roadmap to get started. Next Monday morning, you can begin with the first item on your list. As your confidence builds, you will be able to tackle the next item. If one challenge seems too big, break it down into smaller ones. For example, if walking 30 minutes per day seems like too much, start with 10 minutes per day. If eating slowly and mindfully at every meal seems like too much, start with breakfast only.

If one challenge seems too big, break it down into smaller ones. For example, if walking 30 minutes per day seems like too much, start with 10 minutes per day.

Intermittent Fasting

As discussed in Chapter 1, our bodies can produce from 1 to 4 quarts (1 to 4 liters) of lymph fluid per day. About 50% of this is formed in the gastrointestinal tract and increases after a meal — especially a fatty one. (See Chapter 11: Lymphatics and the Digestion of Dietary Fats for more information.) If you stop eating, you could reduce your lymphatic fluid significantly, but that's not a very practical strategy. Is there a way to fast without starving?

One popular, relatively new weight loss strategy is called intermittent fasting. This involves intentionally restricting food on certain days or during certain times of the day. There are two main methods: the 5:2 and the 16:8. Although neither has been studied in lymphedema, of the two, the 16:8 would be recommended over the 5:2. (Note: neither of these diets is recommended for pregnant women.)

5:2 Intermittent Fasting

In this form of intermittent fasting, you eat a healthy balanced diet 5 days a week and you fast for the other 2 consecutive days (hence the name of this kind of fasting). Some research has been done for cancer patients that shows promising results, including better weight loss and improved sensitivity to insulin.

This is not a method we would recommend for lymphedema patients. Why? Restricting protein for those 2 days could lead to a breakdown of muscle and could lead to more lymphedema (read more about this in Chapter 13: Fluid, Protein and Sodium).

16:8 Intermittent Fasting (Time-Restricted Feeding)

There are 24 hours in a day, and many of us eat during a 12- or 14-hour window. In this type of intermittent fasting, also called time-restricted feeding, we reduce the eating window to 8 hours and increase the fasting to 16 hours (hence the name of this kind of fasting). In time-restricted feeding, you are meeting your protein and fluid needs (water, tea, coffee and other noncaloric liquids are allowed throughout the day), but you are reducing the hours during which the GI tract is working at digesting and absorbing nutrients. The table below shows how you can shorten your eating window and lengthen your fasting window by changing the time of day for your first meal and your last meal.

Typical Eating Pattern vs. Intermittent Feeding

TYPICAL EATING PATTERN	EATING AND FASTING WINDOWS	INTERMITTENT FASTING PATTERN	EATING AND FASTING WINDOWS
7:00 am	Eating begins with breakfast		
12:00	Lunch	11:00 am	Eating begins with late breakfast
3:00 pm	Afternoon snack	3:00 pm	Lunch
7:00 pm	Dinner	7:00 pm	Eating ends with dinner
9:00 pm	Eating ends with evening snack		
Total Eating Window	14 hours		8 hours
Total Overnight Fast	10 hours*		16 hours**

* The fasting hours are from 9:00 p.m. until 7:00 a.m. the following morning, when eating begins.

** The fasting hours are from 7:00 p.m. until 11:00 a.m. the following morning, when eating begins.

Research Review: Time-Restricted Feeding and Weight Loss

In a 2016 study done with 34 men, the 8-hour eating day was compared to the 12-hour eating day. These men, who were all weight training during the 8-week study, lost more body fat with the 8-hour time-restricted feeding day compared with the 12-hour eating day. Both groups maintained their muscle mass. Both groups ate three meals per day and received 100% of their calorie needs.

Sometimes it works out that you are eating only two meals per day.

HOW TO:
Try Intermittent Fasting

1. Before you make any changes to your diet, get some baseline weight and lymphedema measurements for 3 or more days to help you evaluate the effectiveness of the diet. Check out "Self Measurements" on page 26 to see how to do that.

2. To help you plan, look at your daily routine and calculate what your current eating window is on most days. Your goal will be to reduce that window. You don't have to move to a 16:8 ratio right away; you can take gradual steps toward that. Likely, the first step with the biggest impact would be to stop eating after dinner; the second step would be to push back your first meal of the day. It doesn't have to be dramatic on your first morning. It's best to pay attention to your feelings of hunger and fullness.

3. Maintain a routine of weighing yourself and taking lymphedema measurements, and make sure to record the time of your first meal and your last meal so you can calculate the total hours of your eating and fasting windows.

4. Evaluate your results. If you are seeing a reduction in your lymphedema and/or weight loss, you may choose to keep going. Keep in mind that you can eat three to four times during your restricted eating window, but — based on your feelings of hunger and fullness — sometimes it works out that you are eating only two meals per day. If this is the case, be sure you are choosing foods wisely. It's important to plan ahead.

These results were also seen in a 2014 review of both animal and human studies by researchers at California State University. The researchers summarized that time-restricted feeding led to weight loss (though not consistently) and improved metabolic changes (such as lower triglycerides, glucose and LDL cholesterol, and increased HDL), and they called the results of these studies "promising."

Jean's Clinical Experience

When I read the research on time-restricted feeding and weight loss, I begin to speculate that this diet might be beneficial for lymphedema, since eating increases gut lymphatic tissue (GALT) production and this diet allows less time for eating. But try as I might, I could not find any studies on time-restricted feeding and lymphedema, so — at this point — my theory remains speculation. As I have outlined above, there is some evidence to support the theory that this strategy will help with weight loss, and specifically fat loss.

One of my clients gave me this anecdotal report: "I had breast cancer and developed lymphedema in my right arm after treatment. I did my bandaging and worked with a lymphedema therapist, but I noticed a big difference in my arm and shoulder swelling when I cut out my evening snacking. I used to eat at night, mostly out of boredom, but when I stopped, I could see that my arm was much less swollen in the morning."

This single report isn't conclusive evidence, but I think this approach might be worth trying — only the 16:8 time-restricted feeding method (not the 5:2 intermittent fasting method).

The Bottom Line

You can have a positive impact on your lymphedema (and your health) by losing weight. If this is a lifelong struggle for you or seems too onerous, get help! Even if you know what to do to lose weight, working with a registered dietitian can give you fresh ideas, trouble-shooting support and the added accountability that can make *this time* the time that you succeed.

CHAPTER 11

Lymphatics and the Digestion of Dietary Fats

One very important role of the lymphatic system is the role it plays alongside our digestive system. This chapter explores what digestion is and discusses some very interesting research on the different dietary fats, how they are absorbed and how they impact the lymphatic system.

How Does Our Digestive System Work?

The macronutrients in our food — carbohydrates, proteins and fats — are broken down (digested) into their smallest components before they travel through the wall of the small intestine and into the bloodstream. These smallest components are then absorbed into the cells, where they are used for energy and function.

Knowing how the digestive process works, with particular attention to the digestion of fats into fatty acids and how these fatty acids are absorbed, will help you understand how your food can impact your lymphedema.

Digestion takes place in the digestive tract, also known as the gastrointestinal tract (GI tract). It's called the gastrointestinal tract because it includes both the stomach (gastro) and the intestines (small and large intestines), but the GI tract actually includes the full length of the digestive system — from the mouth to the anus. Knowing how the digestive process works, with particular attention to the digestion of fats into fatty acids and how these fatty acids are absorbed, will help you understand how your food can impact your lymphedema.

Mouth

Digestion begins in the mouth, with chewing. This is a form of mechanical digestion, the teeth, jaw and tongue essentially breaking food down into smaller pieces. The food mixes with your saliva, which contains important enzymes (salivary lipase) that begin chemical digestion. The food is formed into a small ball of chewed food (bolus) and then swallowed.

Esophagus and Stomach

The bolus travels down the esophagus, which is essentially a tube, into the stomach. The very acidic stomach in conjunction with digestive enzymes (pepsin and gastric lipase) amps up the chemical digestion. The mixture of partially digested food and acid (called chyme) remains in the stomach until it is gradually released into the small intestine.

Small and Large Intestines

This is the site of the majority of absorption of nutrients from our diet. The body continues to break down the chyme into its smallest nutrient components, and these components continue to travel through the small intestine and exit through the intestine walls to join the bloodstream. This continues into the large intestine until only fiber, sloughed off mucosal cells from the intestines, water and electrolytes remain. The water and electrolytes are the last to be absorbed before the remainder leaves the body in a bowel movement.

Short-, Medium- and Long-Chain Fatty Acids

During digestion, food is broken down into its smallest components. Fats and oils break down into various components, including fatty acids. Fatty acids are chains of carbon atoms and are classified by length: short-chain fatty acids contain fewer than 6 carbons, medium contain between 6 and 12 carbons, and long contain between 13 and 21 carbons. Short- and medium-chain fatty acids exit your small intestine and enter the blood, but long-chain fatty acids hitch a ride through your lymphatic system.

The Lymphatic System Is Part of Digestion and Absorption

Here is a summary of how the lymphatic system plays a part in digestion and absorption.

Short- and Medium-Chain Fatty Acids

Once the chyme is released from the stomach, it enters the first section of the small intestine (the duodenum). At this time, the short- and medium-chain fatty acids are absorbed into the interior of the GI tract (the intestinal lumen) and taken to the portal vein and then onward to the liver.

Long-Chain Fatty Acids

The long-chain fatty acids take a different route. These become emulsified by the bile in the intestines and turn into tiny droplets of fat suspended within liquid. The enzymes pancreatic lipase and colipase then transform the tiny droplets into super-tiny droplets packaged together, called a micelle. The micelles move along to the next two sections of the small intestine, the jejunum and the ileum. As they travel down the intestine, the micelles cling to the bumpy surface (the brush border), where they enter one of the cells of the intestine (an enterocyte). This is where they change form again, this time into a fat-transportation sphere (a chylomicron).

Each tiny protrusion of the brush border (a villus) has a single lymphatic capillary (called a lacteal) running up its center. The chylomicron is moved through the vessels by intestinal rhythmic movements (peristalsis).

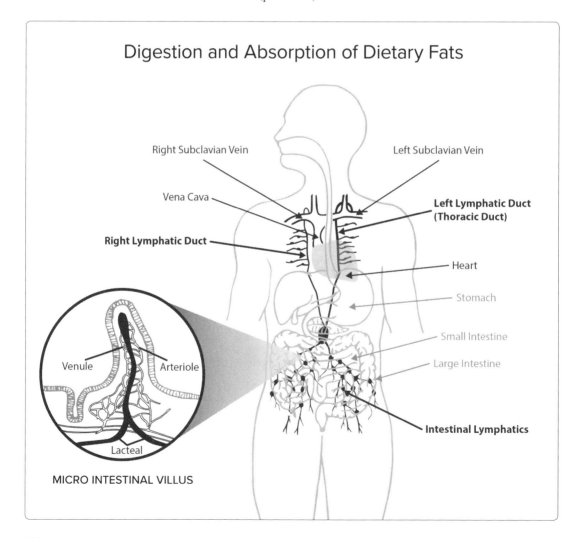

Digestion and Absorption of Dietary Fats

Right Subclavian Vein

Left Subclavian Vein

Vena Cava

Left Lymphatic Duct (Thoracic Duct)

Right Lymphatic Duct

Heart

Stomach

Small Intestine

Large Intestine

Venule — Arteriole

Intestinal Lymphatics

Lacteal

MICRO INTESTINAL VILLUS

Once inside the lymphatic system, the chylomicron becomes a component of the lymphatic fluid; combined, it is known as chyle. Chyle travels up the lymphatic system, which expands into the thoracic duct and then empties into the left subclavian vein. This is where the long-chain fatty acids enter the bloodstream. The blood then delivers the nutrients to the cells where they are needed.

Our bodies can produce 1 to 4 quarts (1 to 4 L) of lymph fluid per day, and 50% of this is formed in the gastrointestinal tract. Now that you appreciate how crucial the lymphatic system is for the transportation and absorption of fats, oils and fat-soluble vitamins (A, D, E and K), it's easy to understand that your lymph fluid will increase after a meal, especially a fatty one.

Bowel Regularity

Constipation is a condition that involves infrequent or hard-to-pass bowel movements. The stool is often hard and dry. Although it's true that what is normal for one person isn't normal for another, you should aim to have a bowel movement that is large, soft and easy to pass. It should resemble a large uncooked sausage in size and consistency. There is no research available to show that constipation increases lymphedema, but some individuals report that constipation can have a negative impact on their lymphedema.

The three main must-haves for healthy bowel movements are fluid, fiber and activity. If you miss one of these, you can develop constipation.

Improving Bowel Regularity

- Before you make any changes to your diet and routine, measure your body weight and take some baseline measurements of your lymphedema to help you evaluate the effectiveness of the diet. Check out "Self Measurements" on page 26 to see how to do that.

- Set a goal to walk 30 minutes every day. If you are not at this level yet, pick a shorter time frame, but commit to daily activity if you are able.

- Aim to drink 64 ounces (2 L) of fluid per day, starting with the morning routine — even if you are not eating at this time. Drink water with your meals and try to reach your fluid goals shortly after the evening meal so that you won't have to use the toilet in the middle of the night.

- Gradually increase the amount of fiber in your diet. Fiber-rich foods include:
  - Whole-grain cereals (read the labels)
  - Whole-grain breads (read the labels)
  - Whole-grain side dishes (such as bulgur, rye, barley, amaranth, wheat berries)
  - Pulse legumes (such as navy, white and black beans; split peas; lentils)
  - Vegetables (such as dark-green leafy greens, peas, broccoli, Brussels sprouts, squash)
  - Fruits (such as berries, pears, figs, prunes, guava)
  - Nuts and seeds (such as flax seeds, almonds, chia seeds)

- Evaluate your results. Following a high-fiber diet, drinking plenty of water and exercising daily is something you should embrace. Even if you do not see any improvement with your lymphedema, it's important for your bowel health.

Research Review: Dietary Fat and Lymphedema

If you change the type or amount of fat in the diet, will it reduce lymphatic fluid volume and therefore improve lymphedema? Below is one animal study and two human studies that explore that question.

STUDY #1

Researchers in Zurich, Switzerland, have studied the effects of a chronic high-fat diet on mice. In a study published in 2014, the researchers noted that lymphatic vessels play an essential role in the intestines' uptake of fats. In their research, they explored what effect a high-fat diet has on lymphatic vessel function. Mice with an impaired lymphatic system were divided into two groups and fed either a normal mouse chow or a high-fat mouse chow. After some time on the diet, the lymphatic vessels were examined under near-infrared imaging. The lymphatic vessels of the mice on the high-fat diet suffered from:

The amount of fat in the diet does impact the lymphatic system in mice — and it may in humans, too.

- Impaired collecting lymphatic vessel function
- Sporadic and less frequent contractions in the lymphatic vessels
- Reduced response to stimulation
- Smaller diameter (meaning they could carry less lymph fluid)

It's interesting to note that the higher the body weight, the worse the lymphatic vessels functioned.

What this study tells us is that the amount of fat in the diet does impact the lymphatic system in mice — and it may in humans, too. Based on these findings, a low-fat diet would appear to be the appropriate nutrition strategy for treating lymphedema in mice. Will this also work for us? On the following pages are two human studies that help to answer this question, but first you need to know about a type of oil that is used in these studies: MCT oil (see box, below).

What Is MCT Oil?

"MCT" stands for "medium-chain triglycerides." This is a manufactured oil, which means it does not occur on its own in nature. To make MCT oil, palm kernel oil and/or coconut oil are fractioned — a process that separates the different fatty acids in the oil. The medium-length fatty acids are separated from the long-chain fatty acids and bottled separately. You can find this oil in some supermarkets, but it's more commonly found in specialty food shops, health food stores and online.

MCT is a clear, light-tasting oil that can be used as a salad dressing or a drizzle on food after cooking; it can also be used for cooking at low temperatures (less than 302°F/150°C). If unopened, the product can be stored in a cool, dry place; once opened, store it at room temperature or in the refrigerator.

STUDY #2

This first of the two human studies is called a case study. As far as research goes, case studies are considered the lowest on the scale in terms of evidence-based credibility, but with so little research available, it's worth sharing.

The study's authors were based in Madrid, Spain, and the case was published in 1994. The case study involved two women with primary lymphedema in their right leg. Patient A was a 30-year-old woman who was put on a weight-loss low-fat diet plus MCT oil. Patient B was put on a low-fat diet plus MCT oil (no weight loss). They followed their diets for 4 months, with monthly follow-ups.

For the diet, they avoided:

- Butter
- Fatty cheese
- Fatty fish
- Fatty meats
- Oils (except for 1 tsp/5 mL of sunflower oil per day)
- Other foods containing significant amounts of long-chain fatty acids

They were allowed to consume MCT oil and they were advised to take a multivitamin-mineral every day.

Results

Here are the results after 4 months on the low-fat diet:

	PATIENT A	PATIENT B
Weight loss	24 pounds (11 kg)	Didn't lose weight (didn't need to)
Reduction in the circumference of the leg without lymphedema	2 inches (5 cm)	No reduction
Reduction in the leg with lymphedema	2.75 inches (7 cm)	1.2 inches (3 cm)

Here is what the diet looked like, by the numbers:

- Calories: not stated
- Carbohydrates: 58% of total calories
- Protein: 22% of total calories
- Fat: 20% of total calories
- MCT oil: 58% of the fat calories

It's hard to know what this diet looked like exactly, with just percentages provided by the researchers, but let's suppose that patient A, who was on a weight-loss diet, received 1200 calories, and let's suppose that patient B, who was on a weight-maintenance diet, received 1800 calories. Here is what their intake of carbohydrate, protein and fat would look like:

NUTRIENTS BY % OF TOTAL CALORIES	1200 CALORIES	1800 CALORIES
Carbohydrates: 58%	174 g	261 g
Protein: 22%	66 g	99 g
Fat: 20%	27 g	40 g
MCT oil: 58% of fat	16 g	23 g

If you are not used to thinking about your nutrition by the numbers, a chart like this can be a bit confusing. It is difficult to know the exact number of grams in the macronutrients that you are consuming without tracking foods in an app or working with a registered dietitian.

Of note is the amount of MCT oil they consumed: 16 grams and 23 grams. Every teaspoon (5 mL) of oil contains 5 grams of fat — translating to 3 tsp MCT oil and $4\frac{1}{2}$ tsp MCT oil (15 mL and 22 mL). Having some sense of the quantities helps us better understand the specifics of their MCT oil intake during the study.

The Bottom Line

Both women experienced a reduction in their leg lymphedema after 4 months on the low-fat diet plus MCT oil. It's important to see that there was still a reduction in lymphedema with the diet change — even without weight loss (as in Patient B).

STUDY #3

This study was conducted by Oliveira and colleagues as a clinical trial, published in 2008 in São Paulo, Brazil. Ten women with upper arm lymphedema following breast cancer surgery, radiation and chemotherapy were included in the study.

Five of the women were in the diet group and the other five served as the control group. Both groups received physiotherapy three times a week for 4 weeks. The control group used corn oil as the main oil in their diet, and the study group used MCT oil as their main oil.

Results

The researchers compared several variables between the two groups. The women who consumed the MCT oil lost 6.8 ounces (200 mL) of arm volume, whereas the corn oil group actually gained $2\frac{1}{2}$ ounces (75 mL) of volume. While this seems very dramatic, the five women

Corn Oil Diet versus MCT Oil Diet		
	CORN OIL DIET	**MCT OIL DIET**
Mean reduction in volume between the arms	Gained 2½ ounces (75 mL)	Lost 6.8 ounces (200 mL)
Mean difference in circumference between the arms	No significant difference in circumference measured at any of the 6 measuring points from the hand to 4 inches (10 cm) above the elbow	Significantly different in one measurement — the point 4 inches (10 cm) below the elbow
Feeling of discomfort (comparing the initial and final values)	Significantly decreased	Significantly decreased
Feeling of arm heaviness (comparing the initial and final values)	Not significantly different	Significantly decreased

who were assigned to the group that received the MCT oil all began the study with greater circumference measurements than the five women in the control group.

The Bottom Line

This was a very small study, but it's interesting that there was an improvement in lymphedema volume with MCT oil and an increase in lymphedema volume with corn oil. Of course, this theory needs to be studied more, but until then, it's reasonable to attempt a low-fat diet plus MCT oil to evaluate if it is helpful for your lymphedema.

It's reasonable to attempt a low-fat diet plus MCT oil to evaluate if it is helpful for your lymphedema.

But … I Thought My Oil Was Healthy

Of all the dietary considerations for lymphedema, this is the most challenging to integrate into a healthy eating plan. This is because the chain length of the fatty acids in your cooking oil is only one measure of the health attributes of the oil — and the chain length is important only in a few instances, lymphedema being one of them.

For example, if you look at the table on page 150, you might think that only MCT oil, coconut oil, palm kernel oil and butter (the options that contain medium-chain fatty acids) are healthy, but there are other factors to consider.

Percentage of Short-, Medium- and Long-Chain Fatty Acids in Various Oils

TYPE OF FAT/OIL	TRIGLYCERIDE CHAIN LENGTH		
	SHORT-CHAIN (FEWER THAN 6 CARBONS)	MEDIUM-CHAIN (6–12 CARBONS)	LONG-CHAIN (13–21 CARBONS)
MCT oil	0	100%	0
Coconut oil	0	64%	36%
Palm kernel oil	0	55%	42%
Butter	5%	7%	89%
Canola oil	0	0	100%
Corn oil	0	0	100%
Flaxseed oil	0	0	100%
Olive oil	0	0	100%
Palm oil	0	0	100%
Safflower oil	0	0	100%
Sesame oil	0	0	100%
Soybean oil	0	0	100%
Sunflower oil	0	0	100%

Source: *Adapted from www.chempro.in and www.chemistryexplained.com.*

Understanding Oils

Oils are made up of fatty acids. These fatty acids are made up of chains of carbon atoms. As we discussed earlier, the length of the chain can be short, medium or long. This is relevant only for people with lymphedema who are interested in reducing the volume of lymphatic fluid and for people who are having difficulty with fat digestion. MCT oil contains just medium-chain triglycerides and this can help with some medical conditions, such as:

- Chyloperitoneum (lymphatic fluid in the peritoneal cavity)
- Gallbladder disease or if removed
- Gastrectomy (stomach removal)
- Pancreatic insufficiency
- Small bowel resection (removal)
- Waldmann's disease

There are other characteristics of oils to consider, such as saturation (saturated or unsaturated) and the presence of a single double bond (monounsaturated) or several double bonds (polyunsaturated). You have likely heard the terms "omega-3" and "omega-6," and this describes the location of the double bond on the fatty acid chain (for example, on the third carbon from the end of the chain, omega 3; or the sixth carbon from the end, omega-6). These have been studied for decades to determine which is the best oil type to reduce the risk of heart disease and inflammation. Here is a quick, super-simplified summary:

Oil Types, Examples and Characteristics

OIL TYPE	OIL EXAMPLES	SIMPLIFIED SUMMARY
Monounsaturated	Olive, high oleic safflower, high oleic sunflower, avocado	Helps raise HDL ("good") cholesterol
Polyunsaturated	Regular safflower, walnut, soybean	When they replace saturated fats, LDL ("bad") cholesterol and triglycerides (TG) improve
Omega-3	Fish, flaxseed, walnut	Essential** and anti-inflammatory
Omega-6	Corn, cottonseed, evening primrose	Essential** but pro-inflammatory
Saturated	Coconut, butter, lard	Raise LDL cholesterol
Trans fats	Partially hydrogenated vegetable oils	Raise LDL and lowers HDL; banned in some countries

Abbreviations: HDL = high-density lipoprotein, a blood fat associated with a reduced risk of heart disease; LDL = low-density lipoprotein, a blood fat associated with an increased risk of heart disease; TG = triglycerides, a blood fat associated with metabolic syndrome (see "Metabolic Syndrome," page 159, for more information)

** Essential fatty acids must be consumed in the diet because the body cannot make them.

Chain Length Matters Only to Some

You may not have heard about chain lengths before, and that's because they are not relevant to the general public. As mentioned earlier, only people with a handful of medical conditions ever need to know about them. In lymphedema, the length of the fatty acid chain makes a difference in the amount of lymphatic fluid that is produced after your meal. What you learned about fats and oils in the past is still true: monounsaturated and polyunsaturated fats — especially omega-3 fatty acids — are healthy, and you need to include a small amount of these in your diet.

Let's look at how medium-chain oils (we'll call them medium-chain triglycerides) compare to long-chain triglycerides.

Monounsaturated and polyunsaturated fats — especially omega-3 fatty acids — are healthy, and you need to include a small amount of these in your diet.

Comparison of Medium- and Long-Chain Triglycerides

MEDIUM-CHAIN TRIGLYCERIDES	LONG-CHAIN TRIGLYCERIDES
100% medium-chain fatty acids	100% long-chain fatty acids
8.3 calories per gram	9.2 calories per gram
Fabricated from coconut and/or palm kernel oil	Naturally occurring in fish, avocado, nuts, seeds, olive and other vegetable oils
Lower smoke point	Higher smoke point
Do not contain essential fatty acids	Contain essential fatty acids
100% saturated fats	Mixture of saturated and unsaturated fats
Can be absorbed directly into the blood via the portal vein	Must enter the lymphatic system for transport into the blood

Source: *Adapted from Parrish, 2017.*

The Case for a Low-Fat Diet

Lymphedema has yet to receive its due in the world of nutritional research. What's presented in this chapter does provide grounds for an argument that a low-fat diet alone or one combined with MCT oil may be helpful for your lymphedema. However, we do know that:

- The physiology of fat digestion shows us that long-chain fatty acids increase lymph volume, while medium-chain triglyceride oil does not.
- Mice on a high-fat diet developed lymphatic vessels that didn't function as well.
- Two small human studies provide us with promising results that indicate a low-fat diet along with MCT oil or a diet with MCT oil as the main oil was helpful for subjects with lymphedema.

What Is a Low-Fat Diet?

The National Institutes of Health (NIH) has determined that 20% to 35% of the calories you consume should come from fat sources in the diet. See the chart opposite to know how much this is.

From this chart, you can see the number of grams of fat in three different calorie levels. A low-fat diet would include approximately 20% of calories from fat. So, for example, if you are following a 1600-calorie diet and wanted to try a low-fat diet, you would need to limit your grams of fat to approximately 36 grams per day. Every teaspoon (5 mL) of fat is 5 grams, so 36 grams of fat would be 7 teaspoons (35 mL). This includes all fats, not just added fats.

Grams of Carbohydrate, Protein and Fat

DAILY CALORIE INTAKE	CARBOHYDRATE* (45%–65%)	PROTEIN (10%–35%)	FAT (20%–35%)
1200 calories	130–312 g	30–105 g	27–47 g
1600 calories	180–416 g	40–140 g	36–62 g
2000 calories	900–1300 g	50–175 g	44–78 g

* The recommended dietary allowance (RDA) for carbohydrate is 130 grams.

Source: *National Institutes of Health; www.nap.edu/read/10490/chapter/8#292.*

HOW TO: Try a Low-Fat Diet

1. Before you make any changes to your diet, measure your body weight and take some baseline lymphedema measurements for 1 week to help you evaluate the effectiveness of the diet. Check out "Self Measurements" on page 26 to see how to do that.

2. Reduce the amount of fat in your diet. In the case study described earlier, researchers advised participants to omit fatty meats, fatty cheese, fatty fish, butter, oils and other fatty foods.

3. Include MCT oil in your diet (see "Guidelines for Using MCT Oil," page 154). Keep in mind that you need to first reduce the current fats in your diet — or at least replace some vegetable oils with MCT oil. Simply adding MCT oil to your regular diet will not be effective.

4. Check out the meal plans on pages 180–182 to see how much fat is considered low-fat for 1500-, 1800- and 2100-calorie diets.

5. Keep doing your lymphedema measurements during the low-fat-diet-and-MCT-oil trial — or have your lymphedema therapist do that for you (if you go often enough for regular monitoring). Continue with your regular lymphedema self-care and don't make any dramatic changes to that.

6. Evaluate your results. If you are seeing a reduction in your lymphedema and/or weight loss, you may choose to keep going. Remember that the body requires essential fatty acids in the diet. If you follow a strict low-fat diet with MCT oil, it is possible that your body could become deficient in essential fatty acids after 3 weeks. A simple solution for this is to include 1 teaspoon (5 mL) per day of a healthy vegetable oil that contains a good ratio of omega-3 to omega-6 fatty acids, such as flaxseed oil, canola oil or hemp oil (you can cook with canola oil, but not with flaxseed or hemp oils).

If you want to try a low-fat diet, follow a diet with around 20% of calories coming from dietary fat and use MCT oil in place of other vegetable oils.

Guidelines for Using MCT Oil

- Begin with a small amount (1 to 2 teaspoons/5 to 10 mL), one to two times per day.
- Increase the amount gradually to prevent any GI side effects (nausea, vomiting, cramping, diarrhea).
- Increase every few days as tolerated.
- Do not exceed 7 tbsp (105 mL) per day, divided throughout your day.
- Do not heat MCT oil over 302°F (150°C) or it can affect the flavor.
- You can fry foods with MCT oil, but only over low heat (if the heat is too high, it may burn and produce an off smell).
- Mix MCT oil into a variety of foods, such as soups, sauces, broths, salad dressings and dips.
- Include 1 tsp (5 mL) of canola, flaxseed or hemp oil in your diet if you are on a low-fat diet plus MCT oil for 3 weeks or more.

The Bottom Line

The lymphatic system and the digestive system are partners in the digestion of our food. Keep both healthy by following a healthy diet. If you want to try a low-fat diet, follow a diet with around 20% of calories coming from dietary fat and use MCT oil in place of other vegetable oils. Remember to measure your lymphedema to see if there is an improvement and have at least 1 teaspoon (5 mL) per day of an oil with omega-3 and omega-6. Don't forget to keep your bowels regular with optimal fiber, fluid and activity.

CHAPTER 12

Reducing Chronic Inflammation

"Currently, lymphatic biology is experiencing an enormous renewal in interest, and the importance of lymphatics in disease is gaining recognition outside of the fields of lymphedema and cancer biology, to now include acute and chronic inflammation."

— Alexander, 2010

As you read in Chapter 10, body weight is very important when it comes to lymphedema. A third and important part of that relationship between body weight and lymphedema is inflammation. Lymphedema, body weight and inflammation are linked and will continue to promote each other unless you break out of this cycle. The relationship looks like this:

Lymphedema, body weight and inflammation are linked and will continue to promote each other unless you break out of this cycle.

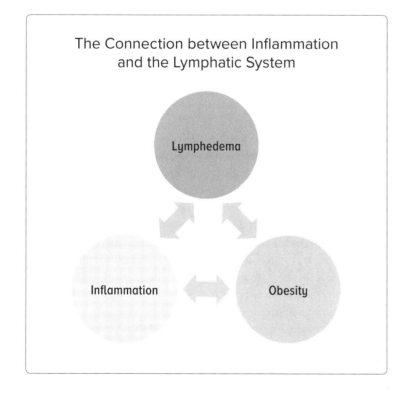

The Connection between Inflammation and the Lymphatic System

Lymphedema

Inflammation

Obesity

What Is Inflammation?

Chronic inflammation continues to dominate not just consumer health books and blogs but also scientific inquiry. But because it is difficult to visualize, it is hard to understand.

There are two types of inflammation: acute and chronic. Chronic inflammation is a condition that is implicated in a variety of diseases, such as heart disease, arthritis and cancer. It's a topic that has been popular for a number of years and it even made the cover of *Time* magazine in February 2004 — the magazine called it the "secret killer." To this day, chronic inflammation continues to dominate not just consumer health books and blogs but also scientific inquiry. But because it is difficult to visualize, it is hard to understand. Here's an analogy that might help you picture what is going on inside your body.

Calling All First Responders

Let's pretend you wake up one day, look out your front window and see a car accident on your street. You call 911 and the first responders come on the scene — the fire truck, the ambulance, the police, the tow trucks — and they all have a job to do. The paramedics provide first aid to the injured person, the firefighters put out any fire and clean up the spilled fuel, the police control the traffic flow, and the tow truck drivers tow away the damaged vehicles. After some time, you look out your window again and your street is back to normal. Think of this as acute inflammation ("acute" means "short-term").

When your body has an injury or infection, the surveillance team of your immune system calls 911 and those cellular first responders come and take care of the scene. You know they are there because of the signs of inflammation: redness, heat, pain, swelling and loss of function. This is acute inflammation in your body and it is a normal, healthy process. After some time, all of these signs subside and things go back to normal.

Let's go back to the scenario on your street. What would happen if those first responders came to the scene but then didn't leave? A lot of looky-loos (you might call them rubberneckers) would be stopping to see what was going on, creating crowded, blocked sidewalks and making it more difficult to pass. The traffic would get backed up behind the accident, which would cause some drivers to become impatient and possibly cause new accidents. There could certainly be some honking and aggression. When garbage day rolls around, the garbage truck wouldn't be able to pass and things would start to get pretty smelly on your street; cockroaches and rats would come on the scene and now your street is in a real state of dis-ease.

Those very same first responders who did their job and left the scene were helpful in the first scenario. But when they stayed where they were no longer needed in the second scenario, they created an environment that allowed new problems to develop. Think of this as chronic inflammation ("chronic" means "long-term").

It's the same in our bodies. Acute inflammation is a very helpful, well-functioning process, but if those same cellular first responders stay in the area, they create a whole new environment that allows disease to take hold and thrive; this includes some types of cancer, heart disease, Alzheimer's disease and rheumatoid arthritis, among others. In very simple terms, you could say that acute inflammation is good (it allows for wound healing and infection control) and chronic inflammation is bad (it creates an environment that allows other health problems to develop).

This environment of chronic inflammation is what exists in your body in the area of your lymphedema.

Inflammation's Role in Disease

A writer for *Science* magazine in 2010 reported that chronic inflammation is one of the most important scientific discoveries in health research in recent years, most notably the fact that inflammation plays a role in not just a few disorders, but in many diseases that cause substantial illness and contribute to early death. Inflammation is involved in at least eight of the top 10 leading causes of death in the United States today.

Inflammation is implicated in the following conditions (among others):

- Alzheimer's disease
- Anxiety
- Asthma
- Cardiovascular disease
- Certain cancers
- Diabetes
- Obesity

- Osteoporosis
- Post-traumatic stress disorder
- Rheumatoid arthritis
- Schizophrenia
- Stroke
- Unipolar and bipolar depression

DID YOU KNOW?

Here are two examples of chronic inflammation leading to the development of new diseases: first, gingivitis increases your risk of heart attack and stroke; second, excess body fat increases inflammatory messengers (called cytokines), which can damage nerves, organs and tissues and eventually lead to diabetes.

What Does Inflammation Have to Do with Lymphedema?

Lymphedema and inflammation are conditions that feed off each other. When inflammation is present, lymphatic function is compromised, which leads to increased lymphedema and obesity — which leads to more inflammation. The diagram on page 158 shows the chain of events that allows this to happen.

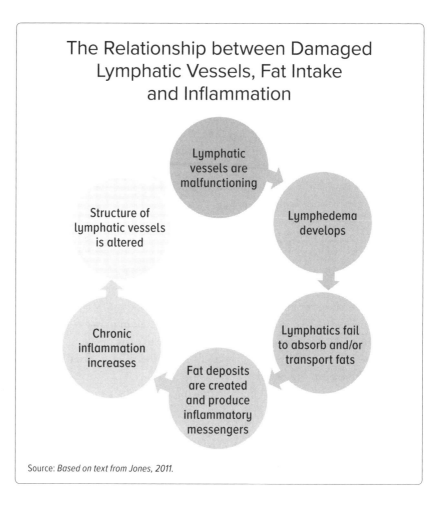

The Relationship between Damaged Lymphatic Vessels, Fat Intake and Inflammation

Lymphatic vessels are malfunctioning

Lymphedema develops

Lymphatics fail to absorb and/or transport fats

Fat deposits are created and produce inflammatory messengers

Chronic inflammation increases

Structure of lymphatic vessels is altered

Source: *Based on text from Jones, 2011.*

Lymphangiogenesis Goes Bad

During inflammation, there is an increase in a process called lymphangiogenesis (lymph-angio-genesis = lymph-vessel-creation). For someone who has lymphedema, this may sound like a good thing — the creation of new lymph vessels, which would allow for new lymphatic pathways to help out the damaged ones.

Unfortunately, the lymphangiogenesis that occurs in an environment of chronic inflammation creates lymph vessels that are either not working properly or not working at all, and during inflammation, cell messengers called cytokines are produced, which damage the lymphatic vessels.

You get the picture: chronic inflammation contributes negatively to your lymphedema, and your lymphedema can cause or worsen inflammation. Let's talk about what you can do about it and how you can reduce chronic inflammation. Spoiler alert: your diet is important.

Metabolic Syndrome

Individuals with lymphatic abnormalities are more prone to developing symptoms of metabolic syndrome. Metabolic syndrome is a collection of at least three of these five symptoms:

- Abdominal obesity
- High blood pressure
- High blood sugar
- High triglycerides
- Low HDL ("good") cholesterol

According to Dietitians of Canada, the recommended diet for metabolic syndrome can be summarized as:

Eat:

- 21 to 38 grams of fiber per day
- Low-fat proteins (such as skinless poultry, lean meat, fish and legumes)

Limit:

- Eggs, liver, shrimp and full-fat dairy (this will limit your dietary cholesterol)
- Deep-fried foods, fast foods and baked goods (this will limit your saturated and trans fats)
- Salty processed foods, such as soups, deli meats and canned foods (this will limit your salt intake)
- Alcohol to 1 serving per day for women and 2 per day for men (note: this does not mean that you can abstain for 6 nights and then binge-drink 7 drinks on a Saturday)

Source: UnlockFood.ca, 2019.

FAQ

Q. If I had cancer and now have lymphedema, will my lymphedema diet also help reduce my risk of my cancer coming back?

A. Just as an anti-inflammatory diet may be helpful for lymphedema, the same may be true for cancer. Cancer cells thrive in an environment of inflammation, and an anti-inflammatory diet is likely very beneficial as an anticancer diet as well. Many of the diet and lifestyle recommendations for an anticancer diet are consistent with the recommendations for lymphedema management, such as losing weight and regular physical activity. Limiting sodium is another recommendation for lymphedema management, and this mirrors the anticancer diet, which focuses on whole foods and limits processed foods (the biggest source of added salt in the Western diet). Although there isn't a specific recommendation that a low-fat diet will reduce cancer risk, if being careful with your fat intake helps you control your body weight, then there will be a benefit for cancer risk.

The Traditional Mediterranean Diet

DID YOU KNOW?

Oleic acid is an omega-9 fatty acid, also known as monounsaturated fat (think olive oil and avocado oil). Sunflowers and safflowers have been developed through traditional plant-breeding techniques, so there are different varieties (four for sunflower and two for safflower). Each of these plants has a high-oleic variety. This means that the oil derived from these is high in heart-healthy oleic acid. Another variety of sunflower and safflower is called high-linoleic. Linoleic acid is an omega-6 fatty acid and, therefore, the type of oil derived from this variety of plant is not recommended as part of an anti-inflammatory diet. If you use safflower or sunflower oil, read the label and choose the high-oleic version.

One dietary pattern that has been studied in multiple scenarios is the traditional Mediterranean diet, with emphasis on the word "traditional" (it's not the souvlaki diet or the spaghetti-and-meatballs diet).

Interest in the traditional Mediterranean diet began with the publication of the now famous Seven Countries Study, in which the diets from seven countries (the United States, Italy, Greece, Japan, Finland, the Netherlands and Yugoslavia) were compared to see which country's population had the lowest rate of heart and blood vessel diseases. The eating pattern of Southern Italy and Greece in the 1950s and 1960s was associated with the lowest rate of cardiovascular disease and death from all causes. Researchers continue to study this diet and it has been confirmed as an anti-inflammatory eating pattern.

In a 2004 study led by scientists from Harvard and with input from Greek scientists, researchers studied the food records of residents of Attica, Greece. Their records were compared to the traditional Mediterranean diet pattern. The greater their adherence to the traditional Mediterranean parameters, the higher their scores:

- Daily consumption of whole grains (rather than refined grains)
- 4 to 6 servings of fruits per day
- 2 to 3 servings of vegetables per day
- Olive oil used as the main oil
- 1 to 2 servings per day of nonfat or low-fat dairy products
- 4 to 6 servings per week of fish, poultry, potatoes, olives, pulses and nuts
- 1 to 3 servings per week of eggs or sweets (decreased the score)
- 4 to 5 servings per month of red meat and meat products (decreased the score)
- 1 to 2 glasses of wine per day (decreased the score)
- Moderate consumption of fat
- Higher intake of monounsaturated fat (such as olive oil) than saturated fats (such as animal products)

The higher the score, the more the individual was considered to be adhering to the traditional Mediterranean diet pattern (researchers simply call this the Mediterranean diet). Once scores were tabulated, they were compared to blood tests and it was found that those who had the highest scores also had the lowest levels of inflammation as measured by blood tests.

Adapting the Traditional Mediterranean Diet for Lymphedema

From the Seven Countries Study, we know that olive oil is a healthy, cardioprotective oil and is part of the Mediterranean diet, as are nuts, seeds and fish. Although the Mediterranean diet is recommended to reduce chronic inflammation, we are faced with a conundrum in the case of lymphedema.

Although healthy, olive oil, nuts, seeds and avocados contain only long-chain fatty acids. As discussed in Chapter 11, only short- and medium-chain fatty acids are absorbed directly into the bloodstream via the portal vein. Long-chain fatty acids travel through the lymphatic system. This means that there is an increase in the amount of lymphatic fluid after you eat foods that contain long-chain fatty acids, which could lead to an increase in your lymphedema. Therefore, even though these fats are part of an anti-inflammatory diet, because you have lymphedema, you may find you have better control of your lymphedema and body weight by limiting your intake.

Although the Mediterranean diet is recommended to reduce chronic inflammation, we are faced with a conundrum in the case of lymphedema.

Not All Long-Chain Fatty Acids Are Equal

There are several different long-chain fatty acids found in vegetable oils. Two of these are the essential fatty acids known as omega-3 and omega-6. According to researchers at the Mid-America Heart Institute in Kansas City in 2018, the type of vegetable oil matters for inflammation. They concluded that vegetable oils rich in omega-3 fatty acids are anti-inflammatory, whereas oils rich in omega-6 fatty acids are pro-inflammatory.

Without specific research to weigh the benefits of a diet low in long-chain fatty acids versus one high in anti-inflammatory oils, perhaps the best recommendation at this time is to continue to include omega-3-rich fish and vegetable oils and nuts in your diet, but to be careful with the portion size: limit your fat intake to 20% or less of calories (see the meal plans on pages 180–182).

In addition, it seems prudent to limit or avoid the oils that contain both long-chain fatty acids (which create more lymph volume) and omega-6 fatty acids (which create more inflammation). In essence, these oils have two strikes against them. Therefore, it would be best to limit the following (listed in order of most inflammatory to least inflammatory, based on the IF Tracker app; see box, page 162):

- Cottonseed oil
- High-linoleic safflower oil (read the label; this is different from high-*oleic*)
- Grapeseed oil
- High-linoleic sunflower oil (read the label; this is different from high-*oleic*)
- Wheat germ oil
- Corn oil
- Soybean oil
- Palm oil
- Walnut oil

In addition, choose lower-fat and lean dairy and meat products.

An Anti-Inflammatory Lymphedema Diet

As we discussed in Chapter 11: Lymphatics and the Digestion of Dietary Fats, your lymphedema may benefit from a low-fat diet and especially one that is low in long-chain fatty acids. You may even choose to include MCT oil, which (if used to replace oils containing long-chain fatty acids) has the potential to reduce your lymphedema — although it could potentially increase inflammation. (If you choose to include MCT oil, make sure the rest of your diet is anti-inflammatory so that your overall diet is a healthy one.) Although such a diet has never been tested in lymphedema, it may well be the best approach, based on current knowledge.

Your lymphedema may benefit from a low-fat diet and especially one that is low in long-chain fatty acids.

As well as following a Mediterranean diet, you may choose to also include some of the top anti-inflammatory foods in your diet. According to the IF Tracker app (see box, below), some of the strongest anti-inflammatory foods are:

- Fish such as mackerel, shad, anchovy, herring and salmon
- Garlic, gingerroot and turmeric
- Chile peppers, spinach, turnip greens and onions
- Acerola cherries and goji berries
- High-oleic sunflower oil, hazelnut oil, canola oil, high-oleic safflower oil and olive oil

The IF Tracker App

Looking for an easy-to-use tool to measure how inflammatory or anti-inflammatory your food choices are? The IF Tracker app uses a mathematical algorithm to assign each food a value representing its anti-inflammatory (positive number) or pro-inflammatory (negative number) strength. Although the tool is based on published research describing the ability of various food components to exert either a pro- or anti-inflammatory effect, the tool itself has not been validated by a research study at the time of publication, meaning we don't know for sure whether it can actually cause a shift in the inflammation in your body. Because of this, you may choose to not focus on the IF Tracker numbers included with the nutrient analysis in each of the recipes in Part 4. Keep in mind: using a tool like this one can still be helpful for accurately tracking your calorie, protein, fat and salt intake — other important aspects of your lymphedema management.

The Bottom Line

Because chronic inflammation is present with lymphedema and because chronic inflammation can make you susceptible to other diseases and make your lymphedema worse, it's best to follow an anti-inflammatory diet. However, because long-chain fatty acids, which are part of the Mediterranean diet, can increase your lymph fluid volume, you should modify the traditional Mediterranean diet to be lower in fat. To do this, your diet should be:

- Rich in vegetables, fruits, whole grains, herbs and spices
- Moderate in omega-3-rich fish
- Moderate in anti-inflammatory nuts and oils
- Moderate in legumes
- Low in meats, sweets and seeds
- Very low in processed foods, salt, fatty meats, high-fat dairy and other fatty foods
- Sparse in inflammatory oils
- Consider using MCT oil in place of oils that contain long-chain fatty acids.

Because long-chain fatty acids, which are part of the Mediterranean diet, can increase your lymph fluid volume, you should modify the traditional Mediterranean diet to be lower in fat.

CHAPTER 13

Fluid, Protein and Sodium

This chapter explores dietary recommendations for fluid, protein and sodium. Although blood vessels and lymphatic vessels have many similarities, they are also different in a number of ways. And the two swelling conditions that can occur in the vessels — edema and lymphedema — are distinct and require different dietary approaches. It's important to determine if your swelling is due to lymphedema or edema. Consult your doctor or health-care specialist for more information and to determine the cause of the swelling if you aren't sure.

Differences between Edema and Lymphedema

In Chapter 1, we discussed the differences between edema and lymphedema (see page 21). It's a long-established medical and nutrition practice to restrict fluid and sodium for edema; in some cases, such as early-stage kidney disease, we also restrict protein.

Comparison of the Diet Recommendations for Various Fluid-Accumulation Disorders				
CONDITION	FLUID RESTRICTION	SALT RESTRICTION	PROTEIN RESTRICTION	DIURETICS
Edema due to congestive heart failure	✔	✔	No	✔
Edema due to kidney disease	✔	✔	Varies**	Varies***
Edema due to liver disease	✔	✔	No	✔
Lymphedema	No	✔	No	No

* See "Are there medications or pills that I can take to treat my lymphedema?" (page 28) for more information.

** Protein restrictions are not recommended for end-stage renal disease but are used in the early stage.

*** Diuretics are not used for end-stage renal disease without urine flow.

Source: Based on data from O'Brien, 2005.

It's important to know what is causing your swelling so that the appropriate nutrition therapy can be used. The chart on page 164 details the differences in dietary therapy.

The chart gives you a quick, at-a-glance view of *what* the recommendations are for fluid, protein and salt, but let's go through the details to help you understand the *why* behind the recommendations.

Drink Sufficient Fluid

When a person has edema related to heart, kidney or liver disease, it is standard protocol for a fluid restriction to be recommended. This also makes intuitive sense: if I have an excess of fluid in my body, then I will drink less to compensate. Why, then, is it not recommended for lymphedema? The reason stems from the difference in the makeup of the edema fluid and the lymphedema fluid. Lymphatic fluid is high in protein and edema fluid is not. This has important implications for the diet prescription.

While no research exists on this specific question, the commonly accepted recommendation around fluid and lymphedema is to drink sufficient fluid throughout the day and not to restrict your fluid intake. The belief is that restricting fluid in your diet will increase the concentration of protein in your lymphatic fluid, and the high protein content will attract more fluid into the lymphedema tissue in an effort to dilute it.

How Much Fluid Do I Need?

There is currently no recommended dietary allowance (RDA) for water, but there are AIs (average intakes) available, and these serve as a general guideline for how much water you should drink. The AI for adults is 2 to 3 quarts (2 to 3 L) per day from fluids. This does not include the fluid content of your food.

Eat Enough Protein

The often-repeated recommendation found on lymphedema websites and in books is not to restrict protein in the diet. While there is also a lack of research on this, the prevailing wisdom is that when you cut back on protein, your body has to look elsewhere for a protein source and will break down your muscle instead. This can lead to weakness and may actually cause more swelling. Albumin, which is a type of protein in the blood, exerts a pressure against the inside of the blood vessel to keep water inside it. When albumin drops, the pressure drops and water can leak out into the interstitial spaces, leading to more lymphedema.

How Much Protein Do I Need?

The RDA for protein is 46 grams per day for women and 56 grams per day for men. A registered dietitian can personalize your protein requirements and may suggest a different target. For example, a dietitian may calculate your protein needs by using either your actual body weight or your ideal body weight, your activity level and your health status.

Restrict Salt Intake

Salt, also known as sodium chloride, is a known water attractor. Although the human trials of a low-sodium diet for the treatment of lymphedema are few and far between, there appears to be a benefit to restricting salt for lymphedema. Let's review the research that does exist and explore the next considerations: Is there harm in recommending a low-sodium diet? Is this a good recommendation for everyone? What should the level of restriction be?

Research Review: Salt Restriction

There are two studies — one in mice and one in humans — that explore the relationship between salt and lymphedema.

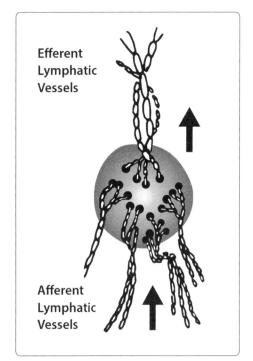

Efferent Lymphatic Vessels

Afferent Lymphatic Vessels

Lymph node close-up; arrows indicate the direction of lymph movement

STUDY #1

The first study, published in 2015 by researchers in Japan, shows that sodium has an effect on lymph nodes. In this study, mice were fed either a normal-salt diet for 9 weeks or a normal-salt diet for 5 weeks followed by a high-salt diet for 4 weeks.

The researchers used microscopes to examine the effect that the high-salt diet had on the individual lymph nodes in the mice. As you can see in the illustration to the left, one lymph node has several lymph vessels coming into it. These are called the afferent vessels ("afferent" means "moving toward"). Filtration takes place within the node and the lymph fluid exits via two larger efferent vessels ("efferent" means "moving away"). The afferent and efferent lymph vessels work as a series of lymphatic pumps to propel the lymph fluid inside the node by tightening and loosening (constricting and dilating).

The mice that received the high-salt diet showed a number of differences (compared to the control group), such as:

- A higher blood pressure
- A decrease in the diameter of the afferent lymphatic vessels
- A decreased pumping activity of the afferent vessels
- An increased frequency of contraction of efferent lymphatics

Although the net effect was that there was no difference in the amount of pumped lymphatic fluid, it does demonstrate that a high-salt diet can affect how lymph vessels function. The higher blood pressure caused by the high-salt diet also had some effects on the lymph node: less lymph fluid was pumped out with each contraction and there was a reduced intensity of pumping.

The authors noted that the different effects of the high-salt diet on the lymphatic vessels of the mice depended on the species, the length of time on a high-salt diet and what part of the body was studied. Although we don't have concrete evidence that a high-salt diet is detrimental for lymphedema, this study suggests that a high-salt diet:

- Increases blood pressure, which reduces the effectiveness of lymph nodes
- Makes the lymph vessels pump less going into the node and pump faster coming out

STUDY #2

You may not be surprised to learn that you have to search all the way back to 1962 to find a study on the effects of a low-sodium diet on lymphedema. The 21 subjects in this study included men and women with congestive heart failure, a buildup of fluid around the heart, and edema in the feet, ankles and legs, as well as three subjects with lymphedema. The study aimed to determine the effectiveness of a liquid formula called Metrecal, which contained only 900 calories and 900 milligrams of sodium per quart (1 L).

Most participants consumed a total of 1000 milligrams of sodium and 1000 calories per day. In other words, this was a very-low-sodium, very-low-calorie diet. This allowed the three lymphedema subjects to lose weight and reduce their lymphedema.

Why talk about this old diet study from the 1960s? It's the only study covering the use of a low-salt diet for lymphedema. What can we learn from it? People lost weight and their lymphedema improved. Of course, you could argue that their lymphedema improved because they lost weight (discussed in Chapter 10). Did the addition of the salt restriction help? This can't be confirmed, because of the way the study was designed, but based on salt's water-attracting properties, a safe bet would be yes. The salt restriction likely helped reduce their lymphedema and it could help your lymphedema, too. (Note: strict calorie and salt restrictions are not sustainable in the long term; like your lymphedema self-management program, you want your diet to be something you can stick with in the long run.)

Is There Harm in Being on a Low-Sodium Diet?

In 2012, physicians from St. Luke–Roosevelt Hospital (now Mount Sinai West) in New York investigated whether low-salt diets were worth the effort, reporting that there were minimal adverse events associated with a low-salt diet. Low blood pressure (hypotension), however, was a possibility. If you are currently taking a blood-pressure-lowering medication, consult with your physician if you notice your blood pressure dropping too much while you're on a salt-restricted diet. (You can tell this is happening if it takes a few seconds to get your equilibrium when you stand up and you experience a few seconds of dizziness; this is called orthostatic hypotension.)

Is the Low-Sodium Diet for Everyone?

The most common application of a low-sodium diet is for people who have high blood pressure (also called hypertension). Some people who are "salt-sensitive" will respond to a low-sodium diet with a drop in blood pressure, while others who are not salt-sensitive will continue to have high blood pressure despite a salt restriction. In a 2012 article, researchers in New York City reported that elderly people, African Americans and obese individuals are more responsive to the blood-pressure-lowering effects of a low-salt diet. For example, a low-salt diet of 1500 milligrams per day will lower the blood pressure of older adults more than younger adults. Not everyone will get the same results for their efforts; the only way to know if you are salt-sensitive or not is to try the diet and monitor your blood pressure results.

Can this salt sensitivity be applied to lymphedema, too? The answer to that question is not known. But you can try a low-sodium diet and see how it works for you. Keep a measurement of your lymphedema and track your salt intake and your symptoms, such as feelings of fullness, pain and heaviness of your lymphedema, to determine if there is any correlation. Keep in mind that if salt sensitivity exists for lymphedema, you may have different results for your low-dietary-salt intake than others you know with lymphedema.

Jean's Clinical Experience

Brenda is a 59-year-old woman with bilateral leg lymphedema. She lost 20 pounds (9 kg) on her own with diet and exercise. Her weight plateaued and she came to see me for diet counseling to get the weight loss going again. Thankfully Brenda had kept excellent food and lymphedema records and I was able to see that her lymphedema worsened on days she'd consumed higher amounts of sodium. I suggested Brenda try a consistent low-sodium diet, which she implemented very diligently. She lost another 20 pounds (9 kg) and her lymphedema improved as well. I would consider Brenda to be salt-sensitive with her lymphedema.

What Level of Salt Restriction Is Recommended?

A variety of medical conditions require a sodium restriction. The estimated average American and Canadian intake of sodium is 3400 milligrams per day, and therapeutic sodium restrictions range from the least strict at 3000 milligrams per day to the strictest at 500 mg per day. However, the lower the level of sodium intake, the more limited the diet becomes. How do you know what level of sodium restriction will be effective for your lymphedema but will not pose an unnecessary burden for you? At this time, with limited data available, it becomes an educated guess to set a general recommendation for lymphedema; trial and error is the best way to determine your individual range.

Try beginning with 2300 milligrams per day maximum. This is based on national guidelines (which are a bit different in different regions). In the United States, the recommendation is that Americans should consume fewer than 2300 milligrams per day of sodium (if you have prehypertension or hypertension, the cap is 1500 milligrams). In Canada, the recommendation is 1000 to 1500 milligrams per day (with a maximum intake of 2300 milligrams). In the United Kingdom, the recommendation is fewer than 2400 milligrams per day. If you are not currently watching your sodium intake and are not reading labels, you are very likely above this value.

For 2000 milligrams of sodium (and lower), it is recommended that you seek the support of your health-care team so they can routinely monitor blood pressure, hydration status, renal function, thirst, fluid intake and weight, and check for signs of pulmonary edema, congestive heart failure or edema.

Top 3 Misconceptions about Salt

1. **"Sea salt or kosher salt is better than iodized table salt because it is 'natural.'"** Regardless of the source of salt, it is the sodium in salt that causes fluid retention.

2. **"Foods high in salt taste salty."** Some foods that are high in salt don't taste very salty because they are mixed with other things, like sugars, that mask the taste. It is important to read food labels to make smart decisions about the foods you eat. Look at the Nutrition Facts table and use it to help keep track of your sodium intake.

3. **"Eating a low-salt diet means I can say goodbye to flavor."** While it may take your taste buds a bit of time to adjust, you will come to appreciate the lower salt concentration in your foods. Try flavoring your foods with lots of different herbs and spices. Food does not have to taste bland.

Source: *Adapted from WHO, 2012.*

➡ **PRO TIP**

The Centers for Disease Control and Prevention reports that the average person consumes an estimated 3400 milligrams of sodium per day — of which 70% comes from restaurant meals and processed foods. Therefore, reducing restaurant meals and processed foods would have the most dramatic impact on your sodium intake.

➡ **PRO TIP**

If you want to aim for 1000 to 1500 milligrams of sodium per day, try setting your daily goal in the middle of the range — about 1200 milligrams, or 400 milligrams per meal. Many of the recipes in this book have less than 400 milligrams of sodium per serving. For those that have more, keep in mind this is a *daily* goal. If you go over in one meal, just try to be under for the next one. Planning ahead makes this much easier.

Top Tips for a Low-Salt Diet

Here's a list of recommendations from top sources, such as the Centers for Disease Control and Prevention (CDC) and Dietitians of Canada, on how to reduce your sodium intake:

DID YOU KNOW?

Salt is sodium chloride. One teaspoon (5 mL) of salt is the same as 2300 milligrams of sodium. "Low-sodium diet" and "low-salt diet" are often used interchangeably, but pay attention because they are different. Tracking your milligrams of sodium is not the same as tracking your milligrams of salt. There are several apps available that you can use to track your sodium, but tracking isn't necessary. If you follow the top tips listed here, your intake will likely be less than 2300 milligrams per day.

1. Eat at home more often and prepare food from scratch.

2. Choose fresh or frozen fruits and vegetables (no sauce or seasoning).

3. Opt for lower-sodium or no-salt-added breads, crackers and cereals.

4. Select fresh or frozen meats, fish and poultry without added saltwater solution (often labeled "seasoned" or "enhanced").

5. Buy lower-sodium cheeses, such as ricotta and mozzarella, and read labels (sodium contents vary widely across different types of cheese).

6. Make your own salad dressings with low-sodium ingredients (see recipes, pages 194–202).

7. Season your food with fresh and dried herbs and spices in place of all types of salt — including sea salt, Himalayan salt, colored salt, iodized salt and seasoned salt.

8. Use homemade stock and make your own soups and chilis (see recipes, pages 204–212).

9. Prepare homemade muffins and cooked grain cereals, such as oatmeal (read the labels on instant cereals).

10. When choosing prepared foods, look for 5% or less sodium and choose low-sodium versions of prepared foods.

    a. Foods that contain 140 milligrams or less per serving are considered low in sodium.

    b. Foods that contain 35 milligrams or less per serving are considered very low in sodium.

11. When you eat out at restaurants, choose smaller portions of salty options.

12. Limit or avoid the following:

    - Soy sauce and teriyaki sauce
    - Salty snacks like chips, pretzels and salted nuts
    - Canned and dehydrated soups, sauces and gravies
    - Processed meat and fish (such as bacon, cold cuts and salted cod)
    - Frozen pizzas and pizza pockets, burritos, burgers and fries
    - Movie theater popcorn
    - Processed cheese slices (American cheese), cheese dip and saltier varieties of cheese
    - Instant puddings and cakes
    - Flavored potato, rice and pasta side dishes

Sodium Food Claims

Here are some sodium-related phrases you may see on food labels:

- Free of sodium/no sodium
- Low in sodium/low salt
- Reduced in sodium/reduced salt
- Lower in sodium/lower in salt
- No added sodium/no added salt

Check the meaning of label claims in your country to make sure you are making smart choices when shopping. In the United States, check the Food and Drug Administration website at www.fda.gov; in Canada, check the Canadian Food Inspection Agency at www.inspection.gc.ca; in the United Kingdom, check the U.K. Government website at www.gov.uk.

What if I Go Over?

It's almost inevitable that you will sometimes exceed your sodium goal. Let's say you are invited to go out for Chinese food. There are a couple of things you can do. First, observe: pay attention to your lymphedema that night and the next morning. Do you feel more swollen? Are your measurements up? This is good feedback, as it tells you how you react to a higher-sodium meal. Second, be proactive. If you know from observation that eating a salty meal will increase your swelling, do extra self-MLD that night or use compression bandages. Finally, plan on low-salt eating for the next day or two to bring the swelling down.

LIVING WITH LYMPHEDEMA

"I haven't made a connection between what I eat and how my lymphedema responds."

The Bottom Line

You do not require a restriction of fluid or protein in your diet to improve your lymphedema, despite the fact that fluid and protein are two of the main components of lymphatic fluid. In fact, you should make sure that you are getting sufficient fluid and protein.

Despite a limited quantity and quality of supporting research, a sodium restriction appears to be a good strategy. Aim for 2300 milligrams per day maximum and monitor both your sodium intake and your lymphedema. Use your data to determine if you are salt-sensitive with your lymphedema. If you are, continue this level of salt restriction as an ongoing strategy.

CHAPTER 14

Supplements

A quick Google or YouTube search of "supplements for lymphedema" reveals several products that are being strongly promoted to treat lymphedema, with talk of great results and testimonials. It makes you want to buy some right away. But you must be careful to first learn about these products before you buy.

A detailed master list of the supplements promoted for use in lymphedema is included in Appendix 3 (page 245). In that section, you will see:

- Common name(s)
- Brand name(s)
- Active ingredient(s)
- What the product is made from
- The type of product
- The purported claim
- The evidence of effectiveness

Do not take any of these supplements without first consulting a health professional trained in the use of these products. Your pharmacist, registered dietitian and physician would all be good resources for you.

Supplements with Promise

The most studied of all the supplements seems to be selenium, and a review of the research on selenium for lymphedema was published as recently as 2016. In that publication, the authors recommended that the research community continue to study selenium for lymphedema and determine the best dosage and how long it can safely be taken.

Other herbs, like Cyclo-3-Fort, show some promise, but there don't appear to be any new studies in the past 20 years. Robuvit and Wobenzym N — each appearing in one study — show some potential. Pycnogenol seems to be more of a preventive supplement than a treatment for lymphedema. Horse chestnut seed extract products such as Venoruton, Paroven, Venostasin, Essaven gel and Somatoline seem more appropriate for lymphedema that is caused by chronic venous insufficiency.

Mixed Results

This mixed bag of results is the reason why these herbal supplements are not part of standard treatment for lymphedema. If anyone is selling you herbal products that "treat lymphedema," this claim is based only on their opinion, possibly on anecdotal evidence (an informal study and testimony) — but not based on published research. Although researchers may theorize that certain products may be beneficial or have biological plausibility, there is no clear winner in this area. If you have an opportunity to be part of a trial that is testing one of these products, you may want to consider it, as such trials can help move these recommendations forward.

CAUTION

Avoid using coumarin and products containing coumarin because of the possibility of liver toxicity.

FAQ

Q. There isn't much research on nutrition for lymphedema. How can I help?

A. You can start by volunteering to be a case study for your lymphedema therapist. Find out if they are willing to write a case report about the changes that you undertake and the results you achieve. Although case reports likely won't change clinical practice right away, they are a way to get the conversation started and could then pique some interest in observational studies — or even clinical trials. Check out the References (page 259) for good articles that explain how to write a case study for publication (Budgell, 2008; Alwi, 2007). You can also check www.clinicaltrials.com to see if there are any trials you could join to help advance the knowledge of lymphedema treatment.

Supplements without Evidence

There are many supplements that have positive Internet endorsements and recommendations but show *zero* evidence of effectiveness for the treatment of lymphedema. So why are there claims that they can help? It could be that research does exist but is extremely difficult to find. It could be that the claim is based more on the active ingredient and how it behaves in laboratory study — rather than in the human body. For example, turmeric contains the active ingredient curcumin, which is an anti-inflammatory, and since lymphedema is a condition involving inflammation, there is an assumption that it will help with lymphedema. Unfortunately, that's not the way the scientific method works. Until the product has been studied in humans with lymphedema, the claims remain conjecture.

A third reason could be that there is evidence that a supplement can help with related conditions, such as edema or chronic venous insufficiency. Lymphatic vessels and blood vessels have some similarities, but they also have some differences (see page 20). So although a supplement may show positive results for the treatment of blood vessel problems, it's not accurate to assume that these positive results will automatically apply to lymphatic vessels.

Another reason supplements are sometimes recommended as a treatment for lymphedema could be because they have a history of use in traditional or folkloric medicine. The recommendation just keeps getting passed down from generation to generation, but it's never actually studied using scientific methods.

Things to Know before You Try a Supplement

It's important to note that although a certain herb may be used in the preparation of a gel, tincture or extract, for example, the manufacturer may be standardizing (making sure an ingredient is present at a specific level) different active ingredients. For example, horse chestnut seed contains many different natural compounds. Research has been done using extract of horse chestnut, but different research teams standardized for different ingredients.

Oxerutins are the main ingredient in the products Venoruton and Paroven, whereas escin is the active ingredient in the products Venostasin and Essaven gel. In addition, one product may be available in different forms; for example, Venostasin is available as a cream for topical use, as a tablet and as a liquid extract. All this needs to be considered when you are deciding what, if any, supplement to try for your lymphedema.

In review of research published between 2004 and 2012 commissioned by the American Lymphedema Framework and the International Lymphedema Framework on botanicals for lymphedema (Poage, 2015), the authors concluded:

- Botanicals may be more effective in cases of lymphedema that arise from venous insufficiency.
- It is best to choose botanical products from Germany, where more testing is done.
- Avoid any product that has not been evaluated by the Food and Drug Administration (the FDA, a U.S.-based public health agency).
- More research is needed to discover if any botanicals can be reliably recommended as a treatment for lymphedema.

FAQ

Q. Should I try a supplement for my lymphedema?

A. The answer to that question depends on you, your lymphedema management and any possible contraindications. Many people are drawn to the idea of using herbal preparations in their care. If this is you, work with a qualified practitioner, measure your lymphedema and track it over time. Evaluate whether the supplement is working, and discontinue use if it is not.

If you have bilateral lymphedema — meaning that both arms or both legs are affected — and you want to try one of the topical creams or gels, do a trial on only one arm or one leg. You need to be very careful when you interpret your results, because sometimes our desire to see positive results can skew our interpretation of our measurements. Book regular sessions with your lymphedema therapist and have them record your measurements (you may want to not tell them which arm or leg is receiving the treatment). Make sure you use a placebo cream when doing a trial; the simple act of massaging a moisturizer into your skin (not the cream itself) could have a positive effect.

It's vital to remember that these supplements should not replace your regular self-care. You must continue with your lymphedema management routine even if you do a cream or supplement trial.

If you are the type of person who is not drawn to using herbal products, don't worry. You do not need to use a supplement. The physical therapies discussed in Part 2 — manual lymphatic drainage, bandaging, compression and exercise — are the gold standard for treatment. On top of these, you can add taping and the dietary therapies discussed in earlier chapters, namely weight loss, salt and fat restriction, anti-inflammatory foods and possibly MCT oil; these have been more thoroughly studied and show fewer concerns about negative side effects.

Questions to Ask Your Health Professional

Here is a list of questions to ask your health professional about herbal products for lymphedema:

- Are there any safety concerns about this product?
- What are the side effects?
- Are there contraindications with drugs, supplements or foods?
- Are there contraindications for diseases or medical conditions?
- What is the recommended dosing and administration?

➡ **PRO TIP**

As you will see in Appendix 3, the names of products can get confusing. That's because many of these supplements come from herbs and they can have more than one common name. They also have a scientific or botanical name and — if the herb has been made into a commercial product (most likely a proprietary blend of some type) — a brand name. In other cases still, the herb is referred to by its active ingredient. If an herb you are interested in isn't listed in the master list in Appendix 3, find out what other names it goes by and check again.

Helpful Resources

If you want to do some research on your own, here is a list of reputable websites that offer details about supplement ingredients and products. Be wary of sites that give you information on a product but are also selling the product. Try to find neutral sources of information; this applies to websites as well as practitioners.

- Memorial Sloan Kettering Cancer Center: www.mskcc.org
- National Institutes of Health, Office of Dietary Supplements: https://ods.od.nih.gov
- Mayo Clinic: www.mayoclinic.org
- Government of Canada Licensed Natural Health Products Database: https://health-products.canada.ca/lnhpd-bdpsnh/index-eng.jsp
- Natural Medicines Comprehensive Database (an excellent resource but requires a subscription): http://naturaldatabaseconsumer.therapeuticresearch.com/home.aspx?cs=&s=NDC

Once you have completed your research and decided on a product to try, make sure you consult with a professional before you begin dosing.

The Bottom Line

There are many self-care and nutrition strategies that you can use to manage your lymphedema. Supplements are not a necessary part of your treatment strategy but could be trialed with the supervision of your health-care team.

CHAPTER 15

Meal Planning

Knowledge is power but action is key — and now is the time to act on your new knowledge. The previous chapters presented a low-fat, low-sodium, anti-inflammatory nutrition plan that will help you lose weight and will be therapeutic for managing your lymphedema. The meal plans in this chapter and the recipes in Part 4 will help you follow the recommendations in that plan. Putting these recommendations into a dietary pattern allows you to visualize what that will look like for your eating routine:

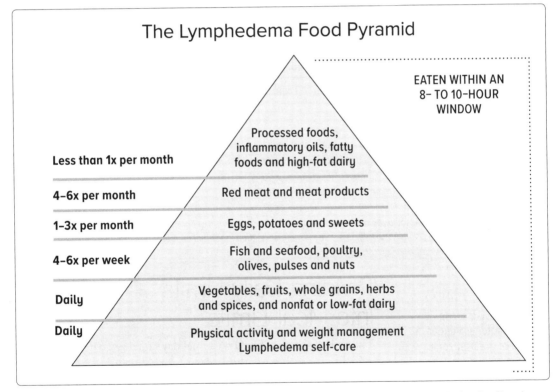

The Lymphedema Food Pyramid

EATEN WITHIN AN 8- TO 10-HOUR WINDOW

Less than 1x per month — Processed foods, inflammatory oils, fatty foods and high-fat dairy

4–6x per month — Red meat and meat products

1–3x per month — Eggs, potatoes and sweets

4–6x per week — Fish and seafood, poultry, olives, pulses and nuts

Daily — Vegetables, fruits, whole grains, herbs and spices, and nonfat or low-fat dairy

Daily — Physical activity and weight management Lymphedema self-care

This pyramid is based on Chrysohoou 2004, and the IF Factor.

It's best to implement these recommendations over time, rather than all at once. Get to know your lymphedema, what helps it and what makes it worse. Measure your lymphedema and observe how it responds to changes in your diet. For example, does your lymphedema respond to a low-salt diet, a low-fat diet, a plant-based anti-inflammatory diet, and/or by limiting your eating window? Maybe all of the above. Knowing what helps you will empower you as you manage your lymphedema in the long term.

Recipe Selection Criteria

Based on the information presented in the previous chapters, these are the criteria for selecting the recipes in Part 4:

CRITERION	AMOUNT	RATIONALE
Weight-reducing	Customized for individual needs*	Weight loss promotes reduction in lymphedema
Low-fat	20% of calories**	Long-chain fatty acids increase lymphatic fluids and inflammation
Anti-inflammatory	A food's anti-inflammatory ranking according to the IF Factor app	Inflammation promotes more lymphedema (and other chronic diseases); diet should be anti-inflammatory
Low-sodium	2300 mg/day*** maximum	Sodium increases the retention of fluid and could increase lymphedema
Sufficient protein	46 g/day adult women 56 g/day adult men[†]	Protein is required to maintain pressure within blood vessels and to maintain fluid balance
High-fiber	21–25 g/day adult women 30–38 g/day adult men[††]	Fiber is anti-inflammatory and promotes regular bowel movements
Added sugars	Fewer than 100 calories (25 g)[†††]	Reducing sugars helps with calorie control and is anti-inflammatory

Dietary Reference Intakes = DRI

* A deficit of 500 calories per day from your usual intake is a standard used in weight-loss research.

** The acceptable macronutrient distribution range for fats is 20% to 35% of total calories.

*** The upper limit for sodium; National Academies, 2018

[†] DRI recommended for protein; National Academies, 2018

[††] DRI recommended for fiber; National Academies, 2018

[†††] American Heart Association recommends a limit of 100 calories (25 g) per day for women and 150 calories (38 g) per day for men (Johnson, 2009); this value is more strict than the DRI of no more than 25% of total calories.

➡ PRO TIP

If you have a sense of the calories in your food or are using one of the calorie-tracking apps, you can set your goal for 500 calories per day less than what you eat now to maintain your weight. This will, in theory, result in a weight loss of about a pound (0.5 kg) a week.

Dividing Daily Limits into Meal Limits

The above values are based on a total day's intake. To determine a guideline for each meal, think about your eating for the day: divide the day into thirds (morning, afternoon and evening meals) and calculate your calories, sodium, protein, fiber and added sugars in thirds. This is customized in the meal plans. Most people eat a small breakfast and a larger meal at the end of the day, so the breakdown goes like this: 25% at breakfast, 35% at lunch and 40% at dinner. In some cases, snacks are included, too. You can see how these numbers look in the meal plans included.

Choosing a Meal Plan for Weight Loss

Chapter 10: Body Weight and Lymphedema detailed two clinical trials that studied the effect of weight loss for lymphedema. Both of the trials used between 1000 and 1200 calories per day for the weight-loss groups. The first trial lasted for 12 weeks and the results were successful. The second trial lasted for 24 weeks and that trial showed that it was difficult for the women assigned to 1200 calories per day to remain on the diet.

Given that lymphedema is a chronic condition and you will need to maintain a healthy way of eating in the long term, for this reason, our meal plan uses 1500 calories. It's important to know that it is very difficult to meet your recommended dietary intakes (RDIs) for vitamins and minerals on a 1200-calorie diet (for example, it's hard to get enough calcium and vitamin D on a limited-calorie diet).

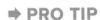

➡ PRO TIP

Talking about calories may work for some people (you know who you are), but it's not for everyone. Your eating doesn't have to be perfect; it just has to be better than it was. So if you used to have two scoops of mashed potatoes and now you have one and a half, that's better than it was. Keep making changes like this and you will see results.

Which Meal Plan Should I Follow?

Everyone's calorie needs are different and will vary by sex, age, activity level, body type and health conditions. Here is a very general guideline to help you determine which of the three meal plans to use as a guide.

MEAL PLAN	SUITABLE FOR
1500 calories	• A woman who is sedentary with a goal to maintain weight • A woman who is rarely to moderately active with a goal to lose weight
1800 calories	• A woman who is very active with a goal to lose weight • A man who is sedentary with a goal to lose weight
2100 calories	• An active woman with a goal to maintain weight • A man who is active with a goal to lose weight

Sample 1500-Calorie Meal Plan

Breakfast

Yogurt bowl made with:
- ¾ cup (175 mL) low-fat plain Greek yogurt
- ⅔ cup (150 mL) blueberries
- ⅔ cup (150 mL) blackberries
- 1½ tsp (7 mL) ground flax seeds (flaxseed meal)
- ⅛ tsp (0.5 mL) ground cinnamon

1 cup of coffee

Morning Snack

1 apple
4 almonds
1 cup of green tea

Lunch

1 serving Squash and Black Bean Chili (page 211)
Salad made with:
- 1 cup (250 mL) green leaf lettuce
- ½ cup (125 mL) chopped red bell pepper
- 1 clementine
- 1 tbsp (15 mL) Golden Salad Dressing (page 202)

¾ cup (175 mL) mixed fruit in juice

Afternoon Snack

1 pear
¾ cup (175 mL) low-fat plain Greek yogurt

Dinner

1 serving Pepper-Crusted Rainbow Trout (page 220)
1 serving Barley with Mushrooms and Caramelized Onions (page 228)
1 cup (250 mL) steamed green beans with a vinaigrette of:
- 1 tbsp (15 mL) lemon juice
- ½ tsp (2 mL) MCT oil
- a pinch each of salt and black pepper

1 grapefruit

How This Meal Plan Helps You Meet Your Daily Goals

	IF RATING	CALORIES	FAT (g)	PROTEIN (g)	FIBER (g)	SODIUM (mg)
TOTALS FOR THE DAY*	Goal: + Actual: +793	Goal: 1500 Actual: 1498	Goal: 33 Actual: 33	Goal: 46 Actual: 83	Goal: 30 Actual: 50	Goal: 2300 Actual: 1305
Morning totals**		341	4	21	13	77
Afternoon totals**		659	14	30	23	717
Evening totals**		498	15	32	14	511

* The fat goal of 33 g is based on 20% of calories and is the maximum intake for the day; the protein goal of 46 g and fiber goal of 30 g are based on the minimum intakes for a woman; the sodium goal of 2300 mg is the maximum intake for the day.

** Morning goals (breakfast + morning snack) are based on 25% of daily total; afternoon goals (lunch + afternoon snack) are based on 35% of daily total; evening goals (dinner) are based on 40% of daily total.

Sample 1800-Calorie Meal Plan

Breakfast

Yogurt bowl made with:
- ¾ cup (175 mL) low-fat plain Greek yogurt
- ½ cup (125 mL) rolled oats
- 1 banana
- 2 tbsp (30 mL) dried cranberries
- 1 tbsp (15 mL) chopped walnuts
- 1 tbsp (15 mL) ground flax seeds (flaxseed meal)

Café au lait made with:
- ¾ cup (375 mL) coffee
- 1 cup (250 mL) skim milk

Morning Snack

1 serving Turmeric Ginger Tea (page 240)

Lunch

1 serving Warm Mushroom and Snow Pea Salad (page 193)

2½-oz (75 g) roasted chicken breast, without skin

1 mango

Afternoon Snack

Yogurt bowl made with:
- ¾ cup (175 mL) low-fat plain Greek yogurt
- ¾ cup (175 mL) grapes
- 8 almonds

Dinner

2 servings Eggplant Tapas (page 186) with 5 low-fat whole wheat crackers

Spaghetti and "meatballs" made with:
- 2 oz (60 g) whole-grain spaghetti
- 1 cup (250 mL) zucchini strips or spirals
- 1 serving Spaghetti Beanballs (page 215)
- 1 serving Garden-Fresh Tomato Sauce (page 230)

¾ cup (175 mL) cherries

How This Meal Plan Helps You Meet Your Daily Goals

	IF RATING	CALORIES	FAT (g)	PROTEIN (g)	FIBER (g)	SODIUM (mg)
TOTALS FOR THE DAY*	Goal: + Actual: +196	Goal: 1800 Actual: 1797	Goal: 40 Actual: 39	Goal: 46 Actual: 109	Goal: 30 Actual: 35	Goal: 2300 Actual: 733
Morning totals**		576	12	33	10	175
Afternoon totals**		586	12	51	9	207
Evening totals**		635	15	25	16	351

*The fat goal of 40 g is based on 20% of calories and is the maximum intake for the day; the protein goal of 46 g and fiber goal of 30 g are based on the minimum intakes for a woman; the sodium goal of 2300 mg is the maximum intake for the day.

**Morning goals (breakfast + morning snack) are based on 25% of daily total; afternoon goals (lunch + afternoon snack) are based on 35% of daily total; evening goals (dinner) are based on 40% of daily total.

Sample 2100-Calorie Meal Plan

Breakfast

Carrot, Mango, Citrus and Ginger Smoothie with Hemp Seeds (page 239)

Morning Snack

Yogurt bowl made with:
- ¾ cup (175 mL) fat-free plain Greek yogurt
- ¾ cup (175 mL) strawberries
- ⅛ tsp (0.5 mL) ground cinnamon

Lunch

1½ servings Red Lentil, Chickpea and Tomato Soup (page 209)
1 serving Roasted Red Pepper Salad (page 195) over 1 cup (250 mL) red leaf lettuce
1 pear

Afternoon Snack

Yogurt bowl made with:
- ¾ cup (175 mL) fat-free plain Greek yogurt
- ¾ cup (175 mL) pineapple
- 1 tsp (5 mL) sunflower seeds

Dinner

1 serving Scotch Salmon (page 219)
¾ cup (175 mL) roasted cubed sweet potato, with a dressing of:
- 2 tbsp (30 mL) fat-free plain Greek yogurt
- 1 tbsp (15 mL) chopped fresh chives
- ½ tsp (2 mL) minced garlic
1 cup (250 mL) steamed broccoli pieces
Fruity green tea smoothie made with:
- ½ cup (125 mL) cold brewed green tea
- ⅔ cup (150 mL) fat-free plain Greek yogurt
- ½ cup (125 mL) fresh or frozen blackberries
- ½ cup (125 mL) fresh or frozen raspberries

How This Meal Plan Helps You Meet Your Daily Goals

	IF RATING	CALORIES	FAT (g)	PROTEIN (g)	FIBER (g)	SODIUM (mg)
TOTALS FOR THE DAY*	Goal: + Actual: +196	Goal: 2100 Actual: 1824	Goal: 47 Actual: 39	Goal: 56 Actual: 117	Goal: 30 Actual: 51	Goal: 2300 Actual: 1097
Morning totals**		384	6	25	11	111
Afternoon totals**		719	13	43	22	627
Evening totals**		721	20	49	18	359

* The fat goal of 47 g is based on 20% of calories and is the maximum intake for the day; the protein goal of 56 g and fiber goal of 30 g are based on the minimum intakes for a man; the sodium goal of 2300 mg is the maximum intake for the day.

** Morning goals (breakfast + morning snack) are based on 25% of daily total; afternoon goals (lunch + afternoon snack) are based on 35% of daily total; evening goals (dinner) are based on 40% of daily total.

The Bottom Line

Lymphedema is a chronic condition, so a short-term diet is not what you are looking for. You want to find an eating pattern that you enjoy, that you can sustain in the long term and that helps (and not worsens) your lymphedema.

PART 4
Recipes for Lymphedema

About the Nutrient Analyses

The recipes for this book were analyzed using the IF Tracker app v3.2, which relies on the USDA nutrient database for calories, protein, fat, carbohydrate, sodium and calcium, plus a proprietary mathematical algorithm to calculate the inflammatory factor (IF). The exceptions are Basic Vegetable Stock (page 204) and Chicken Stock (page 205), which are based on Food Processor SQL and the IF factor for USDA 6700 vegetable broth and USDA 6172 chicken broth. The recipes were input into the IF Tracker app v3.2 by Jean LaMantia, RD, and verified by Monica Reinagel, MS, LDN, creator of the IF Tracker app.

Recipes were evaluated as follows:

- The smaller number of servings was used where there is a range.
- The smaller quantity of an ingredient was used where there is a range.
- The first ingredient listed was used where there is a choice of ingredients.
- A pinch was calculated as ⅛ tsp (0.5 mL).
- Optional ingredients and those that are not quantified were not included in the calculations.
- Marinades were calculated based on 25% absorption of liquid ingredients and 10% retention of solid ingredients (for example, in Bulgogi, page 223).
- Vegetable oil was considered to be 50% soybean oil and 50% canola oil.
- Canned beans that were drained and rinsed were calculated at 41% less sodium than unrinsed canned beans (as per *Today's Dietitian*, 2010).

Each analysis includes the entire recipe divided by the serving size specified and includes the inflammation factor (IF) rating, calories, fat, protein, carbohydrate, sodium and calcium.

At time of publication, the IF rating has not been validated by scientific study. In other words, it is not known with certainty that achieving a positive IF ranking for your total daily food intake will lead to a reduction in your blood inflammation level. While foods and recipes with negative IF ratings can still be considered healthy, for this book, only recipes with positive IF ratings were included. The higher the IF rating, the more anti-inflammatory the recipe is considered to be. (The exception is Chicken Stock, page 205; although it has an IF score of −42, it has other advantages — namely that it's a low-sodium alternative to commercial chicken broths. Adding anti-inflammatory ingredients to this stock will change its rating to anti-inflammatory.)

The IF rating is calculated by taking into account more than 20 different factors that determine a food's inflammatory or anti-inflammatory potential, including:

- Amount and type of fat
- Essential fatty acids
- Vitamins, minerals and antioxidants
- Glycemic index
- Anti-inflammatory compounds

Appetizers, Salads and Dressings

Eggplant Tapas

MAKES 4 SERVINGS

You read in chapter 12 about the anti-inflammatory benefits of the traditional Mediterranean diet, and now you get to taste how delicious that is. If you like spice, add some hot pepper flakes, which amp up both the flavor and the anti-inflammatory punch.

TIPS: You can also cook the eggplant and peppers on the barbecue. Roast until charred, then place in a plastic bag to "sweat" before removing skins.

The eggplant and peppers in this tasty appetizer provide an abundance of vitamins, minerals and antioxidants. You can increase the fiber by serving this nibbler with whole wheat pitas cut into small wedges or with an assortment of fresh vegetables. Any leftovers can be served as sandwiches on whole-grain pitas or crusty whole-grain breadsticks.

- **Preheat oven to 400°F (200°C)**
- **Baking sheet**

1	small eggplant (about 12 oz/375 g)	1
1	medium green bell pepper	1
1	medium red bell pepper	1
2 tbsp	freshly squeezed lemon juice	30 mL
1 tbsp	red wine vinegar	15 mL
1 tsp	olive oil	5 mL
1	clove garlic, minced	1
	Freshly ground black pepper	

1. Place eggplant and bell peppers on baking sheet. Bake in preheated oven for about 30 minutes or until tender and peppers are charred. (Peppers may be finished before eggplant.)

2. Remove skin from peppers and eggplant. Cut eggplant into chunks and cut peppers into thin slices.

3. In a small bowl, combine lemon juice, vinegar, oil, garlic and pepper to taste. Pour over vegetables and stir to coat. Cover and refrigerate for at least 1 hour or up to 24 hours before serving.

This recipe courtesy of Shirley Ann Holmes.

NUTRIENTS PER SERVING	
IF rating	31
Calories	30
Fat	1 g
Protein	1 g
Carbohydrate	5 g
Fiber	2 g
Sodium	2 mg
Calcium	9 mg

Ceviche-Style Crab Cocktail

Jean has made this recipe many times, and it's always a hit. The fresh ingredients will transport you to the shores of a Mexican fishing village. A key to getting the taste just right is picking an avocado that is ready to eat. Serve in small bowls with a fork or spoon, or on firm low-salt whole-grain crackers or tortillas. It's great for a crowd!

TIPS: For ½ cup (125 mL) lime juice, you'll need to purchase 4 or 5 limes.

If not serving right away, wait to add the avocado until just before serving. While the lime juice can delay browning, it won't prevent it entirely.

8 oz	imitation crab pieces	250 g
½ cup	freshly squeezed lime juice	125 mL
2	medium tomatoes, chopped	2
1	small white onion, finely chopped (about ¼ cup/60 mL)	1
1	jalapeño pepper, seeded and chopped	1
¼ cup	fresh cilantro leaves, chopped	60 mL
1	large avocado, cubed	1
	Salt and freshly ground black pepper	

1. If using chunky-style crab pieces, separate them with your fingers; if using finger-style pieces, cut them into ¾-inch (2 cm) pieces.

2. Place crab pieces in a serving bowl and add lime juice, stirring to coat. Stir in tomatoes, onion, jalapeño and cilantro. Add avocado and gently stir just enough to combine without mashing the avocado. Season to taste with salt and pepper. Serve immediately.

NUTRIENTS PER SERVING	
IF rating	69
Calories	133
Fat	8 g
Protein	4 g
Carbohydrate	14 g
Fiber	4 g
Sodium	206 mg
Calcium	20 mg

Fresh Mussels with Tomato Salsa

Serve as hors d'oeuvres or as a salad over lettuce. Mussels are an excellent source of iron and, because of their high level of selenium, they also rank as strong anti-inflammatories.

TIPS: Substitute fresh cilantro for the parsley for a change.

This recipe can also be made with fresh clams.

Prepare and refrigerate mixture early in the day to allow flavors to blend. Spoon into shells a couple of hours prior to serving and keep chilled.

- **Food processor**

24	mussels	24
½ cup	water or dry white wine	125 mL
¾ cup	finely chopped onion, divided	175 mL
1½ tsp	crushed garlic, divided	7 mL
1 cup	coarsely chopped tomato	250 mL
2 tbsp	chopped fresh parsley	30 mL
4 tsp	chopped fresh basil (or ½ tsp/2 mL dried)	20 mL
2 tsp	olive oil	10 mL
¼ tsp	chili powder	1 mL
	Salt and freshly ground black pepper	

1. Scrub mussels under cold running water; remove any beards. Discard any mussels that do not close when tapped.

2. In a saucepan, combine mussels, water, ¼ cup (60 mL) onion and 1 tsp (5 mL) garlic. Cover and steam just until mussels open, about 5 minutes. Discard any that do not open. Let cool, then remove mussels from shells, reserving half of each shell. Place mussels in a large bowl.

3. In food processor, combine the remaining onion and garlic, tomato, parsley, basil, oil, chili powder, and salt and pepper to taste; pulse just until chunky. Do not purée. Add to mussels and stir to mix. Refrigerate until chilled.

4. Divide mussel mixture evenly among reserved half-shells and arrange on a serving plate.

NUTRIENTS PER 1 OF 4 SERVINGS	
IF rating	200
Calories	74
Fat	3 g
Protein	4 g
Carbohydrate	8 g
Fiber	1 g
Sodium	93 mg
Calcium	30 mg

Shrimp and Snow Pea Tidbits

*Medium-sized scallops
would also be delicious for
these very sophisticated
hors d'oeuvres. If serving
cold, prepare and
refrigerate early in the day.*

TIPS: Buy snow peas that are
firm and crisp and have no
blemishes.

To make this recipe even more
anti-inflammatory, use canola,
olive or avocado oil, depending
on your taste preferences.

16	snow peas	16
2 tsp	vegetable oil	10 mL
16	medium shrimp, peeled and deveined, tail left on	16
1 tbsp	chopped fresh parsley	15 mL
1 tsp	crushed garlic	5 mL

1. Steam or microwave snow peas until barely tender-crisp. Rinse with cold water. Drain and set aside.

2. In a nonstick skillet, heat oil over medium heat. Add shrimp, parsley and garlic; cook, stirring, for 3 to 5 minutes or until shrimp are pink, firm and opaque.

3. Wrap each snow pea around a shrimp and fasten with a toothpick. Serve warm or cold.

NUTRIENTS PER 1 OF 4 SERVINGS	
IF rating	46
Calories	69
Fat	4 g
Protein	6 g
Carbohydrate	2 g
Fiber	0 g
Sodium	242 mg
Calcium	32 mg

Beet Salad with Goat Cheese and Toasted Walnuts

Arugula, goat cheese and nuts add wonderful interest and texture to this salad, complementing the flavor of the beets and adding tremendous visual appeal.

TIP: MCT oil is a medium-chain triglyceride, so it doesn't rely on the lymphatic system for transport into the bloodstream; using it in place of olive oil reduces the amount of lymph fluid created after the meal. However, keep in mind that it is more inflammatory than extra virgin olive oil. For more information on MCT oil, see page 146.

3	medium red beets, peeled	3
	Cold water	
⅓ cup	chopped walnuts or pecans	75 mL
1½ tbsp	extra virgin olive oil or MCT oil	22 mL
1½ tbsp	white wine vinegar	22 mL
Pinch	salt	Pinch
	Freshly ground black pepper	
2½ oz	baby arugula	75 g
¼ cup	crumbled reduced-fat goat cheese	60 mL

1. Cut beets in half lengthwise, then cut into ½-inch (1 cm) wedges.

2. Place beets in a saucepan and add enough cold water to cover by at least 1 inch (2.5 cm). Bring to a boil over high heat. Reduce heat and simmer for about 10 minutes or until tender. Drain and let cool.

3. In a small skillet over medium heat, toast walnuts, stirring constantly and being careful not to burn them, for 3 to 5 minutes or until fragrant. Immediately transfer to a bowl and let cool.

4. In a small bowl, whisk together oil, vinegar, salt and pepper to taste.

5. Divide arugula among four plates, top with beets and drizzle with vinaigrette. Garnish with goat cheese and toasted walnuts.

NUTRIENTS PER SERVING	
IF rating	26
Calories	167
Fat	12 g
Protein	5 g
Carbohydrate	9 g
Fiber	3 g
Sodium	182 mg
Calcium	59 mg

Broccoli Slaw with Fresh Mint and Toasted Coconut

Whenever you cook broccoli florets, save the stems for this recipe. You'll love the delightful combination of flavors!

3	broccoli stems, peeled and shredded (about 1½ cups/375 mL)	3
1	green onion (white and green parts), chopped	1
2 tbsp	toasted unsweetened coconut flakes	30 mL
1 tbsp	chopped fresh mint	15 mL
1 tbsp	mayonnaise (regular or light)	15 mL
1 tbsp	plain probiotic yogurt	15 mL
2 tsp	freshly squeezed lemon juice	5 mL
	Salt and freshly ground black pepper	

1. In a large bowl, combine broccoli, green onion, coconut and mint.

2. In a small bowl, whisk together mayonnaise, yogurt and lemon juice.

3. Add mayonnaise mixture to broccoli mixture and stir until evenly combined. Serve cold.

NUTRIENTS PER SERVING	
IF rating	8
Calories	111
Fat	8 g
Protein	3 g
Carbohydrate	8 g
Fiber	2 g
Sodium	78 mg
Calcium	57 mg

Cucumber Raita Salad

Raita is a condiment from the Indian subcontinent. This salad pairs very well with curry dishes or dishes with spice, as it has a cooling effect on your palate.

3 cups	thinly sliced English cucumber, unpeeled (about 1 large)	750 mL
½ tsp	salt	2 mL
½ cup	yogurt cheese (see box)	125 mL
½ tsp	lemon juice	2 mL
¼ tsp	minced garlic	1 mL
¼ tsp	ground ginger	1 mL

1. Place cucumber slices in a large colander and sprinkle with salt. Let stand for 10 to 15 minutes over a large bowl (or in the sink) to drain. Rinse well under cold water. Pat dry and transfer to a bowl. Set aside.

2. In a separate bowl, combine yogurt cheese, lemon juice, garlic and ginger. Add to cucumbers, tossing gently to coat. Chill before serving.

This recipe courtesy of Erna Braun.

Yogurt Cheese

To make 1 cup (250 mL) yogurt cheese, use 2 cups (500 mL) plain low-fat yogurt (Balkan-style, not stirred, made without gelatin). Line a sieve with a double thickness of paper towel or cheesecloth. Pour yogurt into the sieve and place over a bowl. Cover well with plastic wrap and refrigerate for at least 2 hours. Discard liquid and keep in an airtight container in the refrigerator for up to a week.

If you want to drain overnight, use 3 cups (750 mL) yogurt to get 1 cup (250 mL) yogurt cheese. The longer you drain the yogurt, the tarter it becomes.

Yogurt cheese can be used in a variety of dips and dressings.

NUTRIENTS PER SERVING	
IF rating	11
Calories	22
Fat	0 g
Protein	2 g
Carbohydrate	3 g
Fiber	0 g
Sodium	56 mg
Calcium	30 mg

Warm Mushroom and Snow Pea Salad

MAKES 4 TO
6 SERVINGS

A warm, earthy salad like this really satisfies your palate. This dish can be enhanced by using fresh wild mushrooms.

TIP: Look for water chestnuts in the canned vegetable aisle or Chinese food section of the grocery store. They have a crisp texture and add a nice crunch to any salad. Although they have the word "nuts" in their name, water chestnuts are actually an aquatic tuber, and they're very low in fat. They are a good source of vitamin B_6, an important vitamin for the immune system.

VARIATION: Green beans are an excellent substitute for the snow peas.

2 tsp	olive oil	10 mL
1½ tsp	crushed garlic	7 mL
1	medium onion, sliced	1
1 lb	mushrooms, sliced	500 g
8 oz	snow peas	250 g
4 tsp	balsamic or rice vinegar	20 mL
½ cup	water chestnuts, drained and chopped	125 mL
	Lettuce leaves	
4 tsp	freshly grated Parmesan cheese	20 mL

1. In a nonstick skillet, heat oil over medium heat. Add garlic and onion; cook, stirring, until softened, about 5 minutes.

2. Add mushrooms and cook, stirring, just until liquid is released; pour off liquid. Add snow peas and cook, stirring, until tender-crisp, about 2 minutes.

3. Stir in vinegar and water chestnuts; cook for 1 minute.

4. Line a serving platter with lettuce leaves and mound salad over top. Sprinkle with cheese.

NUTRIENTS PER SERVING	
IF rating	138
Calories	111
Fat	3 g
Protein	7 g
Carbohydrate	16 g
Fiber	4 g
Sodium	46 mg
Calcium	72 mg

Sweet Pepper Salad with Red Pepper Dressing

Red pepper is an anti-inflammatory superstar! Although many people believe all vegetables in the nightshade family are inflammatory, this seems to be true only for a minority of people with arthritis who experience more joint pain after ingesting solanine, an ingredient in nightshades. Unless you are one of these people, you can eat red peppers with confidence, knowing that they are anti-inflammatory.

TIPS: Double the recipe for the red pepper dressing and save half to serve as a wonderful side sauce for fish or chicken.

Prepare the dressing up to a day ahead. Stir well and pour over salad just prior to serving.

• **Food processor**

2 cups	chopped red, green or yellow bell peppers	500 mL
1 cup	chopped cucumber	250 mL
1 cup	cherry tomatoes, cut into quarters	250 mL
½ cup	chopped red onion	125 mL
½ cup	chopped celery	125 mL

Dressing

2 tbsp	finely chopped red onion	30 mL
¼ cup	finely chopped red bell pepper	60 mL
1 tbsp	lemon juice	15 mL
2 tsp	red wine vinegar	10 mL
1 tbsp	water	15 mL
2 tbsp	olive oil	30 mL
½ tsp	crushed garlic	2 mL
½ tsp	Dijon mustard	2 mL
2 tbsp	chopped fresh parsley	30 mL
	Salt and freshly ground black pepper	

1. In a salad bowl, combine bell peppers, cucumber, tomatoes, onion and celery.

2. *Dressing:* In food processor, combine onion, red pepper, lemon juice, vinegar, water, oil, garlic, mustard, parsley, and salt and pepper to taste; process until combined.

3. Pour dressing over salad and toss to combine.

NUTRIENTS PER SERVING	
IF rating	183
Calories	111
Fat	7 g
Protein	2 g
Carbohydrate	10 g
Fiber	3 g
Sodium	26 mg
Calcium	30 mg

Roasted Red Pepper Salad

MAKES 6 SERVINGS

For a beautiful presentation, arrange pepper slices on a round platter with their edges overlapping in a circular pattern. Garnish with a large sprig of fresh basil in the center. For a little added spice, sprinkle with a dash of cayenne pepper and crushed garlic.

TIPS: Keep roasted red peppers in your freezer and you can make this salad anytime.

Throughout much of the year, red peppers tend to be expensive. Before buying, weigh peppers of equal size in your hand and choose the lighter ones. Heavier peppers have more seeds, which you end up paying for but not eating.

6	roasted red bell peppers (see box), each cut into 6 strips	6
1 tbsp	balsamic or red wine vinegar	15 mL
2 tsp	olive oil	10 mL
2 tbsp	chopped fresh basil (or 1 tsp/5 mL dried), optional	30 mL
	Freshly ground black pepper	

1. Arrange peppers in the bottom of a shallow serving dish.

2. In a small bowl or measuring cup, whisk together vinegar and oil; drizzle over peppers. Sprinkle with basil (if using). Season to taste with pepper. Chill for at least 1 hour before serving.

Roasting Peppers

Preheat barbecue grill (you can broil in the oven as well, but it's easier and less messy on the barbecue and you can enjoy the outdoors). Place several peppers on the grill and cook until the skins turn black. Keep turning the peppers until the skins are blistered and black. Place the roasted peppers in large stockpot with a lid. The steam will make them sweat, so the skin will be easier to peel off. Let peppers cool, then remove stems, seeds and skin.

NUTRIENTS PER SERVING	
IF rating	97
Calories	40
Fat	2 g
Protein	1 g
Carbohydrate	6 g
Fiber	1 g
Sodium	220 mg
Calcium	11 mg

Best Bean Salad

Canned beans are a time-saver and work very well in this dish. Rinsing has been shown to remove 41% of the sodium from canned beans. To reduce the sodium even more, you can soak and cook dried beans to use in this recipe.

TIPS: Be sure to wash cilantro thoroughly, as it often contains a lot of grit.

Using MCT oil in place of the olive oil would reduce the amount of long-chain fatty acids but would increase the inflammatory effect.

2	large tomatoes, chopped	2
1	can (19 oz/540 mL) mixed bean medley, drained and rinsed	1
¼ cup	finely sliced red onion	60 mL
¼ cup	chopped fresh cilantro	60 mL
2 tbsp	chopped fresh basil	30 mL
Dressing		
1	clove garlic, minced	1
¼ tsp	hot pepper flakes	1 mL
¼ tsp	freshly ground black pepper	1 mL
Pinch	salt	Pinch
1½ tbsp	extra virgin olive oil	22 mL
2 tsp	balsamic vinegar	10 mL
1 tsp	freshly squeezed lemon juice	5 mL

1. In a medium bowl, combine tomatoes, beans, onion, cilantro and basil.

2. *Dressing:* In a small bowl, whisk together garlic, hot pepper flakes, black pepper, salt, oil, vinegar and lemon juice.

3. Pour dressing over bean mixture and toss gently to coat. Cover and refrigerate for at least 1 hour, until chilled, or for up to 1 day.

This recipe courtesy of dietitian Lucia Weiler.

NUTRIENTS PER SERVING	
IF rating	34
Calories	122
Fat	5 g
Protein	5 g
Carbohydrate	16 g
Fiber	4 g
Sodium	196 mg
Calcium	45 mg

Salmon Salad with Peanut Lime Dressing

MAKES 8 SERVINGS

This recipe also works well with tuna or other tasty fish. The dressing is great as a marinade or for stir-fries, and it keeps well for days in the refrigerator. Eating salmon and other fatty fish twice a week is a good way to make sure you are getting enough omega-3s in your diet.

TIPS: If you wish, you can use canned salmon or tuna and skip step 1.

In place of vegetable oil, you could use equally neutral-tasting canola oil, which is more anti-inflammatory.

	Nonstick cooking spray	
8 oz	skinless salmon, cut into ½-inch (1 cm) cubes	250 g
2 cups	halved snow peas	500 mL
6 cups	well-packed romaine lettuce, washed, dried and torn into bite-size pieces	1.5 L
2 cups	sliced red bell peppers	500 mL
1 cup	sliced baby corn cobs	250 mL
½ cup	chopped fresh cilantro or parsley	125 mL

Dressing

3 tbsp	lime juice	45 mL
2 tbsp	peanut butter	30 mL
2 tbsp	water	30 mL
2 tbsp	liquid honey	30 mL
1 tbsp	soy sauce	15 mL
1 tbsp	vegetable oil	15 mL
2 tsp	sesame oil	10 mL
1½ tsp	minced garlic	7 mL
1 tsp	minced ginger	5 mL

1. Heat a nonstick skillet sprayed with cooking spray over high heat. Add salmon cubes and cook, turning often, for 2½ minutes or until fish flakes easily when tested with a fork. Set aside.

2. Blanch snow peas in boiling water or microwave for 1 minute or until tender-crisp. Refresh in cold water and drain.

3. In a serving bowl, combine romaine, salmon, snow peas, red peppers, baby corn and cilantro, tossing gently.

4. *Dressing:* In a small bowl, whisk together lime juice, peanut butter, water, honey, soy sauce, vegetable oil, sesame oil, garlic and ginger.

5. Pour dressing over salad and toss gently to coat.

NUTRIENTS PER SERVING	
IF rating	286
Calories	163
Fat	9 g
Protein	8 g
Carbohydrate	13 g
Fiber	3 g
Sodium	172 mg
Calcium	30 mg

Salade Niçoise

This salad is named for the French city of Nice, located on the French Riviera, and has all the hallmarks of Mediterranean cuisine: olives and olive oil, fresh vegetables, herbs and seafood.

TIPS: Fresh tuna, either grilled or broiled, is fabulous in place of the canned tuna.

In place of vegetable oil, you can use canola oil, which is more anti-inflammatory.

You can prepare the salad and dressing early in the day and toss them together just before serving.

4 oz	green beans, trimmed	125 g
4 cups	torn leaf lettuce	1 L
2	small potatoes, peeled, cooked and chopped	2
1 cup	chopped tomatoes	250 mL
¾ cup	chopped red bell pepper	175 mL
½ cup	sliced red onion	125 mL
2	anchovies, minced	2
1	can (7 oz/213 g) water-packed tuna, drained and flaked	1
½ cup	black olives, pitted and sliced	125 mL
¼ cup	chopped fresh dill (or 1½ tsp/7 mL dried dillweed)	60 mL
2 tbsp	chopped fresh parsley	30 mL

Dressing

2 tbsp	water	30 mL
2 tbsp	red wine vinegar	30 mL
2 tbsp	lemon juice	30 mL
1 tsp	crushed garlic	5 mL
1 tsp	Dijon mustard	5 mL
3 tbsp	vegetable oil	45 mL

1. In a saucepan of boiling water, blanch green beans just until bright green. Drain and rinse with cold water. Drain and set aside.

2. Place lettuce in a large salad bowl. Add green beans, potatoes, tomatoes, red pepper, onion, anchovies, tuna, olives, dill and parsley.

3. *Dressing:* In a small bowl, combine water, vinegar, lemon juice, garlic and mustard. Gradually whisk in oil until combined.

4. Pour dressing over salad and toss gently to coat.

NUTRIENTS PER 1 OF 4 SERVINGS	
IF rating	227
Calories	230
Fat	13 g
Protein	11 g
Carbohydrate	19 g
Fiber	4 g
Sodium	419 mg
Calcium	71 mg

Tuna and Chickpeas with Fresh Lemon Dressing

MAKES 4 SERVINGS

When Jean was working on her Cancer Risk Reduction Guide *(www.cancerriskreductionguide.com) with her business partner and graphic designer, Nesreen Al Hajjar, they would often have lunch together. Jean would make her Beet Salad with Goat Cheese and Toasted Walnuts (page 190), and Nesreen would make this delicious Lebanese Mediterranean salad. Fresh lemon juice is a must for this salad.*

TIP: You can add chopped bell pepper and/or green onions to this salad if you have them on hand.

1	can (5 oz/150 g) water-packed tuna, drained	1
1	can (14 to 19 oz/398 to 540 mL) chickpeas, drained and rinsed	1
1	medium-large tomato, chopped	1
½	English cucumber, chopped	½
¼ cup	fresh parsley leaves, chopped	60 mL
	Juice of 1 large lemon	
2 tbsp	olive oil	30 mL
½ tsp	dried oregano	2 mL
	Salt and freshly ground black pepper	

1. In a large bowl, combine tuna, chickpeas, tomato, cucumber and parsley.

2. In a small bowl, whisk together lemon juice, oil, oregano, and salt and pepper to taste. Pour over tuna mixture and toss gently to coat. Serve immediately.

NUTRIENTS PER SERVING	
IF rating	55
Calories	268
Fat	11 g
Protein	16 g
Carbohydrate	30 g
Fiber	8 g
Sodium	260 mg
Calcium	74 mg

Warm Chicken Salad with Orange Dressing

Chicken, like most other animal products, tends to be an inflammatory food, but making sure to add lots of vegetables as well as herbs and spices to any meat meal helps to make it anti-inflammatory.

TIPS: In place of vegetable oil, you can use canola oil, which has the same mild flavor but is more anti-inflammatory.

The orange juice concentrate gives this dressing an intense flavor. For a lighter taste, omit it.

The dressing can be prepared up to 1 day before and stored in an airtight container in the refrigerator.

Dressing

1 tbsp	chopped fresh tarragon (or 1 tsp/5 mL dried)	15 mL
½ tsp	crushed garlic	2 mL
2 tsp	grated orange zest	10 mL
¼ cup	freshly squeezed orange juice	60 mL
3 tbsp	vegetable oil	45 mL
2 tbsp	light mayonnaise	30 mL
1 tbsp	frozen orange juice concentrate, thawed	15 mL

Salad

1½ cups	snow peas, sliced in half	375 mL
8 oz	boneless skinless chicken breasts, cubed	250 g
1	large head romaine lettuce, torn	1
1 cup	mandarin orange segments	250 mL
½ cup	sliced water chestnuts	125 mL
2 tbsp	chopped pecans	30 mL

1. *Dressing:* In a small bowl, whisk together tarragon, garlic, orange zest, orange juice, oil, mayonnaise and orange juice concentrate until well blended. Set aside.

2. *Salad:* Steam or microwave snow peas just until tender-crisp. Drain and place in a salad bowl.

3. Place chicken in a saucepan and add just enough water to cover; bring to a boil over high heat. Reduce heat to low, cover and simmer for 2 to 3 minutes or until chicken is no longer pink inside. Drain chicken and add to snow peas.

4. Add lettuce, oranges and water chestnuts to salad bowl. Add dressing and toss to coat. Sprinkle with pecans.

NUTRIENTS PER SERVING	
IF rating	13
Calories	174
Fat	10 g
Protein	10 g
Carbohydrate	11 g
Fiber	2 g
Sodium	72 mg
Calcium	39 mg

Raspberry Basil Vinaigrette

Raspberry, balsamic and tarragon vinegars all add extra zest to dressings. To make your own raspberry vinegar, add fresh or frozen raspberries to rice vinegar or white wine vinegar; let stand at room temperature for several days. Strain and bottle. Making your own dressings enables you to reduce your sodium intake, as bottled dressings are typically quite high in sodium.

TIP: To vary the taste of vinaigrette dressings, try experimenting with the many kinds of vinegar now available, such as balsamic, herb-flavored or rice vinegar.

½ cup	water	125 mL
2 tbsp	raspberry vinegar	30 mL
1	small clove garlic, crushed	1
1 tsp	cornstarch	5 mL
1 tsp	chopped fresh basil (or ½ tsp/2 mL dried)	5 mL
½ tsp	poppy seeds	2 mL
¼ tsp	grated lemon or orange zest	1 mL
Pinch	salt	Pinch
1 tsp	olive oil	5 mL

1. In a small saucepan, combine water, vinegar, garlic and cornstarch. Cook over medium heat for about 2 minutes or until thickened. Remove from heat and let cool.

2. In a small bowl, combine basil, poppy seeds, lemon zest, salt and oil. Stir in vinegar mixture. Cover and refrigerate for at least 1 hour before using.

This recipe courtesy of Erna Braun.

NUTRIENTS PER 1 TBSP (15 ML)	
IF rating	11
Calories	9
Fat	1 g
Protein	0 g
Carbohydrate	0 g
Fiber	0 g
Sodium	37 mg
Calcium	4 mg

Golden Salad Dressing

This dressing is Jean's go-to for practically every salad. If you've never used nutritional yeast before, look for it in health food stores or in the health food or baking section of the supermarket. It gives food an umami flavor that is often compared to Parmesan cheese. For this recipe, purchase flaked yeast (not ground) and choose a brand that is fortified with vitamins B₁₂ and D, for additional nutritional benefit.

TIPS: Be careful when working with this dressing, and wipe up any spills quickly, as the turmeric will stain.

Look for flaxseed oil in the dairy case at the supermarket (not with the other vegetable oils), as it needs to be kept refrigerated.

2	cloves garlic, crushed	2
⅓ cup	flaked nutritional yeast	75 mL
1 tsp	ground turmeric	5 mL
¾ cup	flaxseed oil	175 mL
3 tbsp	apple cider vinegar	45 mL
3 tbsp	reduced-sodium tamari	45 mL
	Freshly ground black pepper	

1. In a jar or bowl, combine garlic, yeast, turmeric, oil, vinegar and tamari. Seal jar with a lid and shake, or whisk to combine. Season to taste with pepper.

2. Use immediately or store, covered, in the refrigerator for up to 3 days.

NUTRIENTS PER 2 TBSP (30 ML)	
IF rating	78
Calories	99
Fat	10 g
Protein	2 g
Carbohydrate	1 g
Fiber	1 g
Sodium	121 mg
Calcium	1 mg

Soups and Chilis

Basic Vegetable Stock

Using your own homemade stock (often called broth) as a base for homemade soups and stews allows you to reduce your sodium intake, which is especially important during a flare-up of your lymphedema.

TIPS: Adding 1 tsp (5 mL) salt to this stock increases the sodium to 215 mg per cup (250 mL).

To freeze stock, transfer to airtight containers in measured portions (2 cups/500 mL or 4 cups/1 L are handy), leaving at least 1 inch (2.5 cm) headspace for expansion. Refrigerate until chilled, then freeze for up to 3 months. Thaw in the refrigerator or microwave before use.

- **Large (minimum 6-quart) slow cooker (optional)**

8	carrots, coarsely chopped	8
6	stalks celery, coarsely chopped	6
3	onions, coarsely chopped	3
3	cloves garlic, coarsely chopped	3
6	sprigs parsley	6
3	bay leaves	3
10	black peppercorns	10
1 tsp	dried thyme	5 mL
	Salt (optional)	
12 cups	water	3 L

Slow Cooker Method

1. In slow cooker, combine carrots, celery, onions, garlic, parsley, bay leaves, peppercorns, thyme, salt to taste (if using) and water. Cover and cook on Low for 8 hours or on High for 4 hours.

2. Strain and discard solids. Cover and refrigerate for up to 5 days or freeze in an airtight container.

Stovetop Method

1. In a large pot, combine carrots, celery, onions, garlic, parsley, bay leaves, peppercorns, thyme, salt to taste (if using) and water. Bring to a boil over high heat. Reduce heat to low, cover and simmer gently for about 1 hour or until liquid is flavorful.

2. Strain and discard solids. Cover and refrigerate for up to 5 days or freeze in an airtight container.

NUTRIENTS PER 1 CUP (250 ML)	
IF rating	7
Calories	18
Fat	0 g
Protein	1 g
Carbohydrate	4 g
Fiber	1 g
Sodium	23 mg
Calcium	0 mg

Chicken Stock

*It's easy to make
homemade stock instead
of resorting to commercial
stock cubes and powders,
which are loaded with salt.*

TIPS: Adding 1 tsp (5 mL) salt to
this stock increases the sodium
to 289 mg per cup (250 mL).

To freeze stock, see tip,
page 204.

Despite its negative IF rating,
this stock is a good low-sodium
alternative to commercial
chicken stock. When you make
a soup or stew with it, you can
shift the IF factor by adding anti-
inflammatory ingredients, such
as onion and garlic.

VARIATION: *Turkey Stock:*
Substitute raw turkey wings
for the chicken bones, or use
the carcass of a roasted turkey
(cleaned of meat, skin and fat).

3 lbs	chicken bones (such as neck, backbone and wing tips)	1.5 kg
2	carrots, coarsely chopped	2
2	stalks celery, including leaves, chopped	2
1	large onion, chopped	1
½ tsp	dried thyme leaves	2 mL
1	bay leaf	1
	Freshly ground black pepper	

1. Place chicken bones in a large stockpot. Add water to cover (about 10 cups/2.5 L). Add carrots, celery, onion, thyme and bay leaf. Bring to a boil over high heat and skim off fat. Reduce heat to low and simmer, covered, for 2 hours.

2. Strain through a fine-mesh sieve. Season to taste with pepper. Cover and refrigerate for up to 2 days or freeze in an airtight container.

NUTRIENTS PER 1 CUP (250 ML)	
IF rating	−42
Calories	8
Fat	0 g
Protein	0 g
Carbohydrate	2 g
Fiber	1 g
Sodium	11 mg
Calcium	0 mg

Caramelized Onion and Roasted Mushroom Soup

Caramelizing the onions and roasting the mushrooms adds tremendous flavor to this soup.

TIPS: Marsala is a fortified wine (it has brandy or another spirit added to it) made from Sicilian grapes.

Be sure to remove the rosemary and thyme sprigs before serving so that there are no hard woody parts in the soup.

For an elegant first course for your next dinner party, ladle the soup into bowls and top each with 1 slice of toasted whole-grain baguette and 1 tsp (5 mL) freshly grated Parmesan cheese.

- **Preheat oven to 425°F (220°C)**
- **Rimmed baking sheet**

1 lb	mushrooms, quartered	500 g
2 tbsp	canola oil, divided	30 mL
4	sprigs fresh rosemary, divided	4
4	sprigs fresh thyme, divided	4
1 tsp	freshly ground black pepper, divided	5 mL
2 cups	coarsely chopped onions	500 mL
¼ cup	coarsely chopped shallots	60 mL
¼ cup	Marsala wine	60 mL
4 cups	reduced-sodium chicken broth	1 L
1	bay leaf	1

1. Place mushrooms on baking sheet and drizzle with 1 tbsp (15 mL) oil. Add 2 sprigs each of rosemary and thyme. Sprinkle with ½ tsp (2 mL) pepper. Roast in preheated oven, stirring occasionally, for 20 to 25 minutes or until mushrooms are golden brown. Discard rosemary and thyme sprigs. Set mushrooms aside.

2. Meanwhile, in a large pot, heat the remaining oil over medium heat. Add onions and shallots; cook, stirring, for 2 minutes. Reduce heat to low and cook, stirring often, for about 15 minutes or until onions are caramelized (dark golden brown).

3. Add Marsala and deglaze the pot, scraping up any brown bits stuck to the bottom. Add roasted mushrooms, broth, bay leaf and the remaining rosemary, thyme and pepper; increase heat to high and bring to a boil. Reduce heat and simmer for 15 minutes to blend the flavors. Discard rosemary and thyme sprigs and bay leaf.

This recipe courtesy of dietitian Mary Sue Waisman.

NUTRIENTS PER SERVING	
IF rating	167
Calories	126
Fat	5 g
Protein	6 g
Carbohydrate	15 g
Fiber	3 g
Sodium	438 mg
Calcium	42 mg

Thai-Style Squash Soup

Garlic, ginger, lemongrass, lime and coconut milk bring the flavors of Thailand to your dinner table. If you are lucky enough to have any leftovers, this soup is great as a sauce over grilled fish, chicken or pork.

TIPS: Using canola oil in place of vegetable oil will make this recipe more anti-inflammatory.

This recipe is best when squash is in season. You can often find chopped butternut squash in the produce section of the supermarket.

If you can't find wild lime leaves locally, substitute grated lime zest (3 leaves = the zest of 1 lime).

If you choose to prepare this recipe in a slow cooker instead of on the stovetop (see box, page 210), complete step 2 in the slow cooker, then follow the remainder of the method here. Heat on High for about 20 minutes after adding the coconut milk and lime leaves.

NUTRIENTS PER SERVING	
IF rating	225
Calories	164
Fat	12 g
Protein	3 g
Carbohydrate	14 g
Fiber	2 g
Sodium	310 mg
Calcium	64 mg

- **Preheat oven to 350°F (180°C)**
- **Blender or immersion blender**

1	head garlic	1
1 tbsp	olive oil	15 mL
2 tbsp	vegetable oil	30 mL
1	onion, finely chopped	1
2 tbsp	finely minced gingerroot	30 mL
2 tbsp	finely minced lemongrass	30 mL
1	large butternut squash, peeled, seeded and diced	1
3¼ cups	reduced-sodium chicken broth	800 mL
1	can (14 oz/398 mL) light coconut milk	1
	Salt and freshly ground black pepper	
4	wild lime leaves (optional)	4

1. Cut top off head of garlic to expose the cloves. Place on a small piece of foil wrap. Drizzle with olive oil. Cover with foil and bake in preheated oven for 30 minutes or until cloves are soft.

2. Meanwhile, in a large saucepan, heat vegetable oil over medium heat. Add onion, ginger and lemongrass; cook, stirring, until tender, about 5 minutes. Add squash and broth; bring to a boil. Reduce heat to low, cover and simmer for 30 minutes. Remove from heat. Squeeze roasted garlic into soup, making sure not to get any skin in soup.

3. Working in batches, transfer soup to blender (or use an immersion blender in the pot) and purée on high speed until smooth.

4. Return soup to saucepan (if necessary) and stir in coconut milk. Season to taste with salt and pepper. Add lime leaves (if using). Heat over low heat for 10 minutes or until heated through and lime flavor infuses soup.

This recipe courtesy of Eileen Campbell.

Curried Sweet Potato Soup with Broccoli and Fried Ginger

MAKES 6 SERVINGS

For this soup, the condiments really make the difference. The cilantro, green onion and fried ginger aren't just pretty toppings — they really make this soup pop!

TIP: If you purchase the broth, a 32-oz (900 mL) container is the perfect size — no need to add more broth or water.

- **Immersion blender**

5 tsp	canola oil, divided	25 mL
1	medium onion, chopped	1
1	large clove garlic, minced	1
1 tsp	minced gingerroot	5 mL
1½ tbsp	curry powder	22 mL
1 tsp	ground turmeric	5 mL
⅛ tsp	freshly ground black pepper	0.5 mL
4 cups	cubed peeled sweet potato (about 1 large)	1 L
4 cups	Basic Vegetable Stock (page 204) or reduced-sodium ready-to-use vegetable broth	1 L
4 cups	broccoli florets (about 1 large crown)	1 L
3 tbsp	julienned gingerroot	45 mL
½ cup	fresh cilantro leaves, roughly chopped	125 mL
¼ cup	chopped green onions (green part only)	60 mL
1 cup	low-fat plain probiotic yogurt	250 mL

1. In a large pot, heat 2 tsp (10 mL) oil over medium heat. Add onion and cook, stirring, for 3 to 4 minutes or until softened. Stir in garlic, minced ginger, curry powder, turmeric and pepper; cook for 1 minute or until fragrant.

2. Stir in sweet potato and broth; bring to a boil over high heat. Reduce heat and boil for about 10 minutes or until sweet potato is soft.

3. Using immersion blender, pulse to blend about two-thirds of the soup, leaving some pieces whole.

4. Stir in broccoli and boil gently for 8 to 10 minutes or until tender.

5. Meanwhile, in a small skillet, heat the remaining oil over medium-high heat. Add julienned ginger and cook, stirring, for 5 to 8 minutes or until golden and crispy. Immediately transfer to a plate lined with a paper towel.

6. Ladle soup into bowls and top with cilantro, green onions, fried ginger and a dollop of yogurt.

NUTRIENTS PER SERVING	
IF rating	256
Calories	169
Fat	5 g
Protein	5 g
Carbohydrate	27 g
Fiber	5 g
Sodium	139 mg
Calcium	143 mg

Red Lentil, Chickpea and Tomato Soup

MAKES 4 SERVINGS

When you are in the mood for a warm, comforting soup, this full-flavored vegetarian option should be on your list. Because of its heartiness, you won't miss having meat on your plate, and one serving provides 14 grams of protein, which is equivalent to 2 oz (60 g) meat.

TIPS: Flaxseed oil is not often used for cooking, as it can tolerate only a low heat. But in this recipe, the oil is heated for only a short time. Look for flaxseed oil in the dairy case at the supermarket (not with the other vegetable oils), as it needs to be kept refrigerated. If you prefer, you can substitute olive or canola oil.

Leftover chickpeas can be stored in an airtight container in the refrigerator for up to 1 week and in the freezer for up to 6 months.

NUTRIENTS PER SERVING	
IF rating	91
Calories	257
Fat	6 g
Protein	14 g
Carbohydrate	40 g
Fiber	9 g
Sodium	225 mg
Calcium	107 mg

- **Bullet blender with the extra-tall cup**

2 tsp	cumin seeds	10 mL
2 tsp	hot pepper flakes	10 mL
1 tbsp	flaxseed oil	15 mL
1	red onion, sliced and rings separated	1
¾ cup	dried red lentils, rinsed	175 mL
1	can (14 oz/398 g) whole tomatoes, with juice	1
3 cups	water	750 mL
½	can (14 to 15 oz/398 to 425 mL) chickpeas, drained and rinsed	½
1½ tsp	dulse granules	7 mL
¼ cup	chopped fresh cilantro, divided	60 mL
¼ cup	plain Greek yogurt	60 mL

1. In a large saucepan, heat cumin seeds and hot pepper flakes over medium-high heat for 1 minute or until seeds are just starting to pop. Add oil and heat until shimmering. Add onion and cook, stirring, for 5 minutes or until translucent.

2. Stir in lentils, tomatoes and water; bring to a boil, stirring often. Reduce heat and simmer for 7 to 10 minutes or until lentils are just tender. Transfer to a large bowl and let cool.

3. Working in batches if necessary, add lentil mixture to the extra-tall cup. Twist the extractor blade onto the cup to seal. Blend for 20 seconds or until smooth.

4. Return soup to the pan and stir in chickpeas and dulse. Cook over medium-low heat, stirring occasionally, for 5 minutes or until heated through. Stir in 3 tbsp (45 mL) cilantro.

5. Spoon into bowls, top each with a dollop of yogurt and garnish with the remaining cilantro.

Cilantro Bean Soup

MAKES 8 SERVINGS

A great way to use up fresh cilantro, this flavorful purée needs only a multigrain roll with hummus to make it a filling lunch or dinner. A high-fiber soup choice!

TIPS: You can substitute canola oil for the vegetable oil to make this soup even more anti-inflammatory.

Pack this for lunch on a chilly day with half a multigrain bagel, yogurt and fruit.

You do not have to purée this soup if you would rather have it chunky.

VARIATIONS: Use black beans, red kidney beans or chickpeas in place of the white beans.

Substitute sweet potato for the regular potato, for a change of taste.

- **Blender or immersion blender**

1 tbsp	vegetable oil	15 mL
2	onions, chopped	2
1 cup	diced carrots	250 mL
½ cup	diced celery	125 mL
½ tsp	ground cumin	2 mL
½ tsp	ground coriander	2 mL
1	can (19 oz/540 mL) white beans, drained and rinsed (about 2 cups/500 mL)	1
1	tomato, seeded and chopped	1
3½ cups	reduced-sodium chicken or vegetable broth	875 mL
1 cup	roughly chopped fresh cilantro	250 mL
1 cup	diced peeled potato	250 mL
	Salt and freshly ground black pepper	
	Additional chopped fresh cilantro (optional)	

1. In a large saucepan, heat oil over medium heat. Add onions, carrots and celery; cook, stirring, until softened, about 5 minutes. Stir in cumin and coriander; cook for 1 minute.

2. Stir in beans, tomato, broth, cilantro, potato, and salt and pepper to taste; bring to a boil. Reduce heat, cover and simmer for 25 minutes or until vegetables are just soft. Remove from heat.

3. Working in batches, transfer soup to blender (or use an immersion blender in the pot) and purée on high speed until smooth. Return to pot and reheat, if necessary.

4. Ladle into bowls and garnish with cilantro, if desired.

This recipe courtesy of Eileen Campbell.

Making Soup in a Slow Cooker

Get all of your ingredients ready the night before and sauté any vegetables that need precooking. For soups that include ground meat, cook the meat separately from the vegetables, making sure it is completely cooked. Refrigerate the cooked vegetables and meat in separate airtight containers. In the morning, add all the ingredients to the slow cooker and set to Low. In about 8 hours, give or take a bit, you'll arrive home to the tantalizing aroma of freshly made soup.

NUTRIENTS PER SERVING	
IF rating	75
Calories	130
Fat	2 g
Protein	7 g
Carbohydrate	22 g
Fiber	7 g
Sodium	266 mg
Calcium	69 mg

Squash and Black Bean Chili

Flavored with cumin and chili powder, with a hint of cinnamon, this luscious chili makes a fabulous weeknight meal. This is a generous serving. Just add a tossed green salad, relax and enjoy.

TIPS: If you are halving this recipe, be sure to use a small (1½- to 3½-quart) slow cooker.

Add the chipotle pepper if you like heat and a bit of smoke.

Step 1 can be completed up to 2 days ahead. Cover and refrigerate until you're ready to proceed with step 2.

- **Medium to large (3½- to 5-quart) slow cooker**

1 tbsp	olive oil	15 mL
2	onions, finely chopped	2
4	cloves garlic, minced	4
1 tsp	dried oregano	5 mL
1 tsp	ground cumin	5 mL
½ tsp	salt	2 mL
1	3-inch (7.5 cm) cinnamon stick	1
1	can (28 oz/796 mL) no-salt-added tomatoes, with juice, coarsely chopped	1
2 cups	cooked black beans	500 mL
4 cups	cubed peeled butternut squash (1-inch/2.5 cm cubes)	1 L
2 tsp	chili powder	10 mL
2	green bell peppers, finely chopped	2
1	can (4½ oz/127 mL) chopped mild green chiles	1
1	finely chopped chipotle pepper in adobo sauce (optional)	1
	Finely chopped fresh cilantro leaves	

1. In a skillet, heat oil over medium heat. Add onions to pan and cook, stirring, until softened, about 3 minutes. Add garlic, oregano, cumin, salt and cinnamon stick and cook, stirring, for 1 minute. Add tomatoes and bring to a boil. Transfer to slow cooker.

2. Add beans and squash to slow cooker, stirring well. Cover and cook on Low for 6 hours or on High for 3 hours, until squash is tender.

3. Scoop a little of the cooking liquid into a small bowl and add chili powder. Stir until dissolved. Add to slow cooker along with bell peppers, green chiles and chipotle pepper (if using). Cover and cook on High for 20 minutes or until bell pepper is tender. Discard cinnamon stick. When ready to serve, ladle into bowls and garnish with cilantro.

NUTRIENTS PER SERVING	
IF rating	240
Calories	209
Fat	3 g
Protein	9 g
Carbohydrate	40 g
Fiber	11 g
Sodium	193 mg
Calcium	98 mg

Cranberry Chicken Chili

MAKES 10 SERVINGS

This is a great recipe for a crowd, and a nice change from beef chili. The cranberries and green peppers float, making a colorful presentation that's perfect for the festive season. Serve with a multigrain roll and fruit salad for a satisfying meal.

TIPS: You can substitute canola oil for the vegetable oil to make this chili even more anti-inflammatory.

If you cannot find fresh or frozen cranberries, use dried ones for a sweeter taste.

Instead of dirtying a cutting board or food processor, use kitchen scissors or a knife to chop canned tomatoes right in the can.

The longer you cook this dish, the more the flavor develops. However, be careful not to cook it so long that the beans disintegrate.

1 tbsp	vegetable oil	15 mL
3	stalks celery, chopped	3
2	cloves garlic, chopped	2
1	large onion, chopped	1
8 oz	mushrooms, sliced	250 g
1	large green bell pepper, chopped, divided	1
1½ lbs	lean ground chicken or turkey	750 g
2	bay leaves	2
2 tbsp	chili powder	30 mL
1 tbsp	chopped fresh parsley	15 mL
1 tsp	hot pepper flakes	5 mL
1	can (19 oz/540 mL) stewed tomatoes, chopped or mashed	1
1	can (19 oz/540 mL) dark red kidney beans, drained and rinsed	1
½ cup	vegetable juice (optional)	125 mL
1 cup	fresh or frozen cranberries	250 mL

1. Heat a large saucepan over medium heat. Add oil and swirl to coat pan. Add celery, garlic, onion, mushrooms and half the green pepper; cook, stirring, until tender. Remove vegetables to a plate.

2. Add chicken to saucepan and cook, breaking it up with a spoon, until no longer pink. Drain off any fat and return to saucepan. Stir in sautéed vegetables, bay leaves, chili powder, parsley and hot pepper flakes; cook for 5 minutes. Add tomatoes and cook for 5 minutes. Stir in beans, being careful not to break them. Dilute mixture with vegetable juice if too thick. Reduce heat and simmer for 30 minutes or longer (see tips), adding vegetable juice if necessary.

3. Add cranberries and the remaining green pepper just before serving.

This recipe courtesy of dietitian Judy Jenkins.

NUTRIENTS PER SERVING	
IF rating	51
Calories	198
Fat	8 g
Protein	17 g
Carbohydrate	17 g
Fiber	5 g
Sodium	319 mg
Calcium	64 mg

Mains and Sides

Lentils Bolognese

This easy recipe is a great vegetarian take on a traditional Italian dish. Serve on top of whole wheat spaghetti and sprinkle with freshly grated Parmesan cheese.

1 cup	dried brown or red lentils	250 mL
2 cups	water	500 mL
1	bay leaf	1
2 tbsp	olive oil	30 mL
2	cloves garlic, crushed	2
1	onion, finely chopped	1
1 cup	sliced mushrooms	250 mL
1 cup	chopped canned tomatoes	250 mL
1	can (5½ oz/156 mL) tomato paste	1
1	apple, diced	1
½ cup	apple cider vinegar	125 mL
1 tsp	dried oregano	5 mL
	Juice of 1 lemon	

1. In a medium saucepan, bring lentils, water and bay leaf to a boil over high heat. Reduce heat to medium and cook for about 20 minutes or until lentils are soft. Drain and rinse; discard bay leaf.

2. In a large saucepan, heat oil over medium heat. Add garlic, onion and mushrooms; cook, stirring, until softened, about 5 minutes. Add cooked lentils, tomatoes, tomato paste, apple, vinegar, oregano and lemon juice; bring to a boil. Reduce heat, cover and simmer for 45 minutes.

This recipe courtesy of Elaine Bass.

NUTRIENTS PER SERVING	
IF rating	37
Calories	164
Fat	4 g
Protein	8 g
Carbohydrate	26 g
Fiber	5 g
Sodium	195 mg
Calcium	39 mg

Spaghetti Beanballs

These vegetarian beanballs are a great alternative to traditional meatballs. Served with tomato sauce, they make a hearty addition to a bowl of spaghetti or a whole-grain roll.

TIPS: For a gluten-free version, use gluten-free panko (Japanese bread crumbs) or gluten-free cracker crumbs in place of the wheat germ.

Serve with Garden-Fresh Tomato Sauce (page 230), over noodles or in a whole-grain roll.

Store beanballs in an airtight container in the refrigerator for up to 3 days or in the freezer for up to 3 months. Let thaw overnight in the refrigerator. Reheat by simmering in tomato sauce for 10 minutes.

- **Preheat oven to 400°F (200°C)**
- **Bullet blender with the tall cup**
- **Baking sheet, lined with foil, foil sprayed with nonstick cooking spray**

1¾ cups	canned soybeans, drained and rinsed	425 mL
½ cup	wheat germ, divided	125 mL
2 tbsp	freshly grated Parmesan cheese	30 mL
1½ tbsp	lightly packed basil leaves	22 mL
1 tsp	onion powder	5 mL
1	clove garlic	1
¼ cup	unsweetened soy milk	60 mL

1. Add soybeans, ⅓ cup (75 mL) wheat germ, Parmesan, basil, onion powder, garlic and soy milk to the tall cup. Twist the extractor blade onto the cup to seal. Blend for 30 seconds or until coarsely combined.

2. Using your hands, roll mixture into 1½-inch (4 cm) balls. Roll balls in the remaining wheat germ. Arrange balls, 1 inch (2.5 cm) apart, on prepared baking sheet.

3. Bake in preheated oven for 12 to 15 minutes or until firm and hot in the center and wheat germ is lightly browned.

NUTRIENTS PER SERVING	
IF rating	9
Calories	122
Fat	5 g
Protein	10 g
Carbohydrate	12 g
Fiber	4 g
Sodium	166 mg
Calcium	120 mg

Broccoli and Mushroom Stir-Fry with Tofu

For great results every time, you can't go wrong with adding broccoli, mushrooms, ginger and green onions to a stir-fry. Serve over brown rice or quinoa.

1 tbsp	canola oil	15 mL
6	green onions (white and green parts), thinly sliced	6
2	cloves garlic, minced	2
1	1-inch (2.5 cm) piece gingerroot, minced	1
¼ tsp	hot pepper flakes	1 mL
8 oz	extra-firm tofu, cubed	250 g
3 cups	broccoli florets	750 mL
7 oz	cremini or white mushrooms, quartered	200 g
3½ oz	shiitake mushrooms, stems removed, caps sliced	100 g
2 tbsp	reduced-sodium tamari	30 mL
1 tsp	sesame oil	5 mL

1. In a large skillet, heat canola oil over medium heat. Add green onions, garlic, ginger and hot pepper flakes; cook, stirring, for about 2 minutes or until softened.

2. Add tofu and cook, turning, for 5 to 10 minutes or until browned on all sides. Add broccoli, cremini mushrooms and shiitake mushrooms; cook, stirring, for 4 to 5 minutes or until broccoli and mushrooms are tender. Stir in tamari and sesame oil.

NUTRIENTS PER SERVING	
IF rating	211
Calories	120
Fat	5 g
Protein	7 g
Carbohydrate	13 g
Fiber	4 g
Sodium	196 mg
Calcium	150 mg

Tandoori Haddock

Tandoori paste makes an easy marinade for white fish. This Indian-inspired dish can be made quickly for a great weeknight meal. For a balanced meal, serve with rice pilaf and steamed sugar snap peas and Cucumber Raita Salad (page 192).

TIP: Most supermarkets now carry tandoori paste. You can usually find it where Indian and Asian sauces are displayed.

VARIATION: This recipe works well with most firm white fish fillets or steaks, such as halibut or orange roughy, and even salmon. Adjust the broiling time depending on the thickness of the fish.

- **Rimmed baking sheet, lightly greased**

¼ cup	tandoori paste (see tip)	60 mL
¼ cup	low-fat yogurt	60 mL
1 tbsp	freshly squeezed lemon juice	15 mL
4	haddock fillets (about 14 oz/420 g total)	4

1. In a shallow dish, combine tandoori paste, yogurt and lemon juice. Add fish, turning to coat evenly. Cover and refrigerate for 20 to 30 minutes.

2. Meanwhile, preheat broiler, with rack placed 4 inches (10 cm) from the heat source.

3. Place fish on baking sheet and broil for 10 minutes or until fish is opaque and flakes easily when tested with a fork and the top is lightly browned.

This recipe courtesy of Eileen Campbell.

NUTRIENTS PER SERVING	
IF rating	174
Calories	96
Fat	1 g
Protein	17 g
Carbohydrate	4 g
Fiber	1 g
Sodium	576 mg
Calcium	37 mg

Salmon in a Parcel

MAKES 4 SERVINGS

Do you avoid cooking fish because you are worried about the smell it sometimes leaves in the kitchen? In this recipe, the fish is enclosed in foil, and no smell escapes at all.

TIP: The rule of thumb for cooking fish is 10 minutes per inch (2.5 cm) of thickness. The thicker the fish, the longer you need to cook it.

- **Preheat oven to 450°F (230°C)**
- **Rimmed baking sheet**

4	salmon fillets (about 1 lb/500 g total)	1
1	lemon, thinly sliced	1
½ cup	chopped fresh dill	125 mL
1 tbsp	olive oil	15 mL

1. Cut four pieces of foil big enough to completely wrap each piece of fish. Place a salmon fillet in the center of each piece of foil. Top each with lemon slices, sprinkle with dill and drizzle with oil. Fold foil over fish and crimp in the center. Tuck excess foil under, pinching to seal edges. Place foil packets on baking sheet.

2. Bake in preheated oven for about 20 minutes or until salmon is opaque and flakes easily when tested with a fork.

This recipe courtesy of Eileen Campbell.

NUTRIENTS PER SERVING	
IF rating	991
Calories	273
Fat	19 g
Protein	24 g
Carbohydrate	3 g
Fiber	1 g
Sodium	68 mg
Calcium	29 mg

Scotch Salmon

Salmon is such a great source of anti-inflammatory omega-3 fatty acids. Try to eat salmon or other omega-3-rich fish twice a week.

- **Rimmed baking sheet, greased**

1	clove garlic, minced	1
1 tsp	grated gingerroot (optional)	5 mL
⅓ cup	Scotch whisky	75 mL
¼ cup	pure maple syrup	60 mL
1 tbsp	canola or olive oil	15 mL
1 tbsp	reduced-sodium soy sauce	15 mL
4	pieces skinless salmon fillet (about 1 lb/500 g total)	4

1. In a small bowl, combine garlic, ginger (if using), Scotch, maple syrup, oil and soy sauce.

2. Place salmon in a shallow glass or ceramic dish. Pour marinade over fish and let stand at room temperature for 15 to 30 minutes (no longer).

3. Meanwhile, preheat broiler, with rack placed 4 inches (10 cm) from the heat source.

4. Pour marinade into a small saucepan. Place salmon on prepared baking sheet. Broil for 7 to 10 minutes or until fish is opaque and flakes easily when tested with a fork.

5. Meanwhile, bring the reserved marinade to a boil over high heat. Reduce heat and simmer for 3 to 4 minutes or until slightly thickened.

6. Serve salmon topped with sauce.

This recipe courtesy of dietitian Mary Bamford.

NUTRIENTS PER SERVING	
IF rating	960
Calories	367
Fat	19 g
Protein	24 g
Carbohydrate	14 g
Fiber	0 g
Sodium	196 mg
Calcium	33 mg

Pepper-Crusted Rainbow Trout

MAKES 4 SERVINGS

There's nothing like fresh rainbow trout! Whether you're lucky enough to catch it yourself or you pick up fresh fillets from your local fishmonger, rainbow trout is a tasty way to stock up on health-promoting omega-3 fats. Rainbow trout is also sometimes called silver trout or steelhead. It is stocked in the Great Lakes and caught off the Pacific shore. It is a freshwater fish that can adapt to salt water. This simple recipe cooks up hot and tasty, with lots of freshly ground black pepper.

TIPS: Keep your kitchen fan on to quickly remove any excess smoke that may be generated from searing the fish at a high heat.

This seems like a lot of pepper, but it yields a delicious, spicy flavor.

VARIATION: Use salmon or arctic char instead of trout and increase the cooking time in step 3 as necessary.

NUTRIENTS PER SERVING	
IF rating	411
Calories	236
Fat	11 g
Protein	24 g
Carbohydrate	6 g
Fiber	2 g
Sodium	160 mg
Calcium	66 mg

4 tbsp	coarsely ground black pepper	60 mL
¼ tsp	coarse sea salt	1 mL
4	rainbow trout fillets (about 1 lb/500 g total)	4
1 tbsp	canola oil	15 mL
1 cup	dry white wine	250 mL
¼ cup	freshly squeezed lemon juice	60 mL

1. In a large, shallow dish, combine pepper and salt; spread out over bottom of dish. Firmly press trout fillets, flesh side down, into pepper mixture, coating flesh completely (do not coat the skin side). Shake off excess and set aside on a clean plate. Discard any excess pepper mixture.

2. In a large skillet, heat oil over medium-high heat until hot but not smoking. In batches as necessary, place fillets, flesh side down, in skillet. Cover and cook for 1 to 2 minutes or until fish is brown and crispy. Transfer fish to a plate. Repeat with the remaining fillets.

3. Return trout to pan, flesh side up. Reduce heat to medium-low and add wine and lemon juice to the skillet. Cover and cook for 8 to 10 minutes or until fish is opaque and flakes easily when tested with a fork. If pan begins to dry out, add 1 to 2 tbsp (15 to 30 mL) water.

This recipe courtesy of dietitian Michelle Gelok.

Stir-Fried Scallops with Curried Sweet Peppers

MAKES 4 SERVINGS

This is an easy, elegant dish with just a few ingredients. You can adjust the amount of curry powder for those who do not like the dish too spicy. Be careful not to overcook the scallops, as they are delicate.

TIP: This is great served over whole-grain pasta or couscous, quinoa or brown rice.

2 tbsp	curry powder	30 mL
	(or 2 tsp/10 mL mild curry paste)	
1 tbsp	olive oil, divided	15 mL
Pinch	salt	Pinch
1	red bell pepper, julienned	1
1	green bell pepper, julienned	1
1	yellow bell pepper, julienned	1
1 lb	sea scallops, halved horizontally	500 g
½ cup	white wine, apple juice or water	125 mL
1 tsp	dark sesame oil	5 mL
1 tbsp	chopped fresh cilantro	15 mL

1. In a large bowl, combine curry powder, 1 tsp (5 mL) oil and salt. Add scallops and toss to coat.

2. In a wok or a large skillet, heat the remaining oil over medium-high heat. Add scallops and stir-fry for 1 minute. Add red, green and yellow peppers; stir-fry for 1 minute. Add wine and cook, stirring, for 3 to 4 minutes or until scallops are firm and opaque. Stir in sesame oil.

3. Using a slotted spoon, remove scallops and vegetables to a serving bowl. Boil sauce, uncovered, for 3 to 5 minutes or until thickened. Taste and add salt, if needed.

4. Pour sauce over scallops and vegetables and sprinkle with cilantro. Serve immediately.

This recipe courtesy of dietitian Edie Shaw-Ewald.

NUTRIENTS PER SERVING	
IF rating	227
Calories	173
Fat	6 g
Protein	15 g
Carbohydrate	10 g
Fiber	3 g
Sodium	521 mg
Calcium	30 mg

Fusion Chicken

This dish incorporates the tastes of many different cultures, and it tastes even better the second day! Serve over brown rice with steamed cauliflower and a Greek salad.

TIPS: You can substitute canola oil for the vegetable oil to make this even more anti-inflammatory.

If desired, once you've ladled Fusion Chicken onto plates, top each portion with a dollop of low-fat or nonfat plain yogurt and sprinkle with chopped fresh cilantro.

VARIATIONS: For a vegetarian version, replace the chicken breast with chickpeas and the chicken broth with vegetable broth.

If you prefer, replace half of the chicken breasts with boneless skinless chicken thighs.

3 tbsp	all-purpose flour	45 mL
1 tsp	salt	5 mL
½ tsp	ancho chile powder or regular chili powder	2 mL
1 lb	boneless skinless chicken breasts, cut into small cubes	500 g
2 tbsp	vegetable oil (approx.)	30 mL
1 tbsp	mild curry powder	15 mL
4	shallots, sliced	4
2	cloves garlic, minced	2
1	red bell pepper, finely chopped	1
1¼ cups	reduced-sodium chicken broth	300 mL
⅓ cup	golden raisins	75 mL
2 tbsp	tomato paste	30 mL
1 tbsp	freshly squeezed lime juice	15 mL

1. In a large plastic bag, combine flour, salt and chile powder; add chicken and shake to coat.

2. In a large skillet, heat oil over medium-high heat. Add chicken, discarding excess flour. Brown chicken on all sides. Add curry powder and toss to coat chicken; cook for 1 minute or until chicken is no longer pink inside. Remove chicken to a plate and set aside.

3. Add more oil to the skillet, if necessary. Add shallots and garlic; cook, stirring, for 2 minutes. Stir in red pepper, broth, raisins, tomato paste and lime juice. Return chicken to skillet; reduce heat and simmer for 15 to 20 minutes or until chicken is heated through and sauce has thickened.

This recipe courtesy of Tina Profiri.

NUTRIENTS PER SERVING	
IF rating	80
Calories	244
Fat	12 g
Protein	18 g
Carbohydrate	16 g
Fiber	2 g
Sodium	605 mg
Calcium	35 mg

Bulgogi (Korean Barbecued Beef)

This easy beef dish needs to be marinated ahead of time, but it cooks quickly and tastes delicious. Serve over brown rice with stir-fried vegetables or in a whole-grain tortilla with stir-fried vegetables. To keep with the Asian theme, serve wedges of fresh Asian pear or lychees for dessert.

TIP: Marinate and cook extra meat. Let cool, slice and store in the fridge for a fast topper for an entrée salad.

1 lb	thin-cut sirloin steak	500 g
4	green onions, finely chopped	4
2	cloves garlic, crushed	2
1 tbsp	finely grated gingerroot	15 mL
¼ cup	reduced-sodium soy sauce	60 mL
¼ cup	liquid honey	60 mL
1 tbsp	sesame seeds	15 mL
1 tbsp	sesame oil	15 mL

1. Pierce steaks with a fork to allow marinade to penetrate.

2. In a large sealable plastic bag, combine green onions, garlic, ginger, soy sauce, honey, sesame seeds and sesame oil. Add steak, seal bag and toss to coat. Refrigerate for at least 30 minutes or for up to 4 hours. Preheat barbecue grill to medium-high.

3. Remove steak from marinade and discard marinade. Place steak on grill and cook for 2 to 3 minutes per side or until desired doneness. Remove steak to a plate and tent with foil. Let rest for 5 minutes, then slice across the grain into strips.

This recipe courtesy of Eileen Campbell.

NUTRIENTS PER SERVING	
IF rating	9
Calories	227
Fat	14 g
Protein	21 g
Carbohydrate	5 g
Fiber	0 g
Sodium	178 mg
Calcium	25 mg

Honey-Glazed Carrots

There's no reason for food in a lymphedema diet to taste bland. Adding a bit of honey, orange zest and ginger makes these carrots flavorful and delicious.

NUTRIENTS PER SERVING	
IF rating	30
Calories	82
Fat	2 g
Protein	1 g
Carbohydrate	16 g
Fiber	3 g
Sodium	79 mg
Calcium	39 mg

1 lb	carrots, cut into 1-inch (2.5 cm) pieces	500 g
1 tbsp	liquid honey or packed brown sugar	15 mL
½ tsp	grated orange zest (optional)	2 mL
1 tbsp	orange juice	15 mL
2 tsp	butter or margarine	10 mL
½ tsp	ground ginger	2 mL

1. In a medium saucepan over high heat, boil carrots until tender-crisp; drain.

2. Add honey, orange zest (if using), orange juice, butter and ginger. Stir quickly for 2 to 3 minutes or until a glaze forms.

This recipe courtesy of dietitian Lynn Roblin.

Sweet Potato "Fries"

Here's a delicious alternative to french fries — with more nutrients and less fat.

NUTRIENTS PER SERVING	
IF rating	133
Calories	119
Fat	2 g
Protein	2 g
Carbohydrate	23 g
Fiber	3 g
Sodium	63 mg
Calcium	35 mg

- **Preheat oven to 375°F (190°C)**
- **Nonstick baking sheet**

1 lb	sweet potatoes, each cut lengthwise into 6 wedges	500 g
2 tsp	vegetable oil	10 mL
¼ tsp	paprika	1 mL
⅛ tsp	garlic powder	0.5 mL
	Freshly ground black pepper	

1. Place potatoes in a bowl. Add oil, paprika and garlic powder. Season to taste with pepper. Toss to coat. Transfer to baking sheet. Bake for 25 minutes or until tender and golden, turning once.

This recipe courtesy of dietitian Bev Callaghan.

Slow-Roasted Cauliflower

MAKES 8 SERVINGS

Jean's family loves these slow-roasted cauliflower bites so much, they eat them like candy. You can serve them as a side dish or snack.

TIP: Because the cauliflower is roasted at a low heat, MCT oil can be used in this recipe, which is great, as its medium-chain fatty acids don't require the lymphatic system for digestion. If you want to speed up the roasting time by increasing the oven temperature, use olive oil, which is anti-inflammatory and can tolerate higher heat. Either way, your roasted cauliflower will be delicious!

- **Preheat oven to 300°F (150°C)**
- **Baking sheet, lined with parchment paper**

1	head cauliflower, cut into florets	1
1 tbsp	olive oil or MCT oil (see tip)	15 mL

1. In a large resealable bag or bowl, combine cauliflower and oil; shake or toss to evenly coat. Spread out in a single layer on prepared baking sheet.

2. Bake in preheated oven for 1 hour. Flip pieces over and bake for 30 minutes or until browned on both sides.

NUTRIENTS PER SERVING	
IF rating	32
Calories	35
Fat	2 g
Protein	2 g
Carbohydrate	4 g
Fiber	2 g
Sodium	24 mg
Calcium	17 mg

Stir-Fried Chinese Greens

This wonderful side dish for grilled fish or chicken is easy to prepare — and even easier if you wash and cut the vegetables the night before. For a full meal, add stir-fried tofu and serve over brown rice.

TIP: You can substitute canola oil for the vegetable oil to make this even more anti-inflammatory.

1 tbsp	vegetable oil	15 mL
1	Spanish onion, sliced lengthwise into thick slices	1
1	green bell pepper, julienned	1
1	head bok choy, cut into chunks (about 4 cups/1 L), white stalks and green leaves separated	1
1 cup	broccoli florets	250 mL
½ cup	water	125 mL
1 tbsp	hoisin sauce or your favorite stir-fry sauce	15 mL
2 tsp	reduced-sodium soy sauce	10 mL
½ tsp	sesame oil	2 mL
1 tbsp	sesame seeds	15 mL

1. Heat a wok or large skillet over medium heat. Add oil and swirl to coat. When oil is hot but not smoking, add onion and stir-fry for 3 minutes. Add green pepper and stir-fry for 2 minutes. Add white stalks of bok choy and broccoli; stir-fry for 2 minutes. Stir in bok choy leaves, water, hoisin sauce and soy sauce; cover and cook for 3 minutes or until broccoli is tender-crisp.

2. Transfer to a serving dish, drizzle with sesame oil and sprinkle with sesame seeds.

This recipe courtesy of Eileen Campbell.

NUTRIENTS PER SERVING	
IF rating	102
Calories	72
Fat	4 g
Protein	2 g
Carbohydrate	8 g
Fiber	2 g
Sodium	140 mg
Calcium	70 mg

Red Beans and Red Rice

Here's a fresh twist on the classic Southern dish of red beans and rice. Bulked up with muscular red rice, this is very hearty — with the addition of salad, it's a meal in itself. The green peas add a burst of color, making this a visually attractive dish that looks good on a buffet. It is particularly tasty as an accompaniment to roast chicken or a platter of roasted vegetables.

TIPS: If you're using chicken stock to cook the rice, you may not need the added salt.

You can cook your own beans or use 1 can (14 to 19 oz/398 to 540 mL) no-salt-added red kidney or small red beans, drained and rinsed.

An IF rating is not available for this recipe because the IF for red rice is unknown.

VARIATION: Substitute brown rice or a mixture of brown rice and wild rice for the red rice.

1 tbsp	olive oil	15 mL
1	onion, finely chopped	1
1	green bell pepper, finely chopped	1
4	stalks celery, diced	4
4	cloves garlic, minced	4
1 tsp	dried thyme	5 mL
½ tsp	salt (see tip)	2 mL
½ tsp	cracked black peppercorns	2 mL
¼ tsp	cayenne pepper	1 mL
1 cup	Wehani or Camargue red rice, rinsed and drained	250 mL
2 cups	water or reduced-sodium chicken stock	500 mL
2 cups	drained, rinsed cooked or canned red beans (see tip)	500 mL
2 cups	cooked green peas	500 mL

1. In a Dutch oven, heat oil over medium heat for 30 seconds. Add onion, bell pepper, celery and garlic; cook, stirring, until pepper is softened, about 5 minutes. Add thyme, salt, peppercorns and cayenne; cook, stirring, for 1 minute.

2. Add rice and toss to coat. Add water and bring to a boil. Reduce heat to low, cover and simmer until rice is tender and most of the water is absorbed, about 1 hour. Stir in beans and peas and cook, covered, until heated through, about 10 minutes.

NUTRIENTS PER SERVING	
IF rating	n/a
Calories	201
Fat	3 g
Protein	8 g
Carbohydrate	37 g
Fiber	6 g
Sodium	203 mg
Calcium	52 mg

Barley with Mushrooms and Caramelized Onions

Caramelized onions and two mushroom varieties add deep, rich flavor to this dish.

TIPS: Hulled barley is a better choice than pearl barley, as it is a whole grain, but it is difficult to find in stores. Another option is pot barley, which is more readily available and is less processed than pearl barley. To use pot barley in this recipe, use the same amount of water and increase the cooking time to close to 1 hour.

Do not let the onions scorch in step 2. If they start to get dark spots, add a little water.

1½ cups	water	375 mL
⅔ cup	pearl barley, rinsed	150 mL
1 tsp	canola or olive oil	5 mL
1 cup	chopped onion	250 mL
1 tsp	butter or non-hydrogenated margarine	5 mL
2 cups	sliced white mushrooms	500 mL
1½ cups	shiitake mushroom caps (about 3 oz/90 g)	375 mL
2 tsp	minced garlic	10 mL
1½ tsp	reduced-sodium soy sauce	7 mL
¼ tsp	freshly ground black pepper	1 mL
1½ tsp	minced fresh thyme	7 mL

1. In a medium saucepan with a tight-fitting lid, bring water to a boil over high heat. Stir in barley. Cover and return to a boil. Reduce heat to low and simmer, stirring occasionally, for 30 to 35 minutes or until barley is tender. Remove from heat and drain off any excess liquid.

2. In a large skillet, heat oil over medium heat. Add onion and stir to coat with oil. Cook, stirring often, for 10 minutes or until golden brown. Transfer to a bowl and set aside.

3. Return skillet to medium heat and melt butter. Add white mushrooms, shiitake mushrooms and garlic; cook, stirring, for 4 to 5 minutes or until tender. Return onions to pan. Stir in cooked barley, soy sauce, pepper and thyme.

This recipe courtesy of Compass Group Canada.

NUTRIENTS PER SERVING	
IF rating	43
Calories	124
Fat	2 g
Protein	4 g
Carbohydrate	24 g
Fiber	5 g
Sodium	54 mg
Calcium	20 mg

Sauces, Dips and Drinks

Garden-Fresh Tomato Sauce

This fresh and inviting tomato sauce is the perfect accompaniment to your favorite whole-grain pasta dish. Making your own sauce allows you to control the ingredients, especially the amount of salt and added sugar.

TIPS: If you are able to find high-oleic sunflower oil, that will provide more anti-inflammatory omega-3 fatty acids. You can also substitute olive oil, which is an easy find.

If you prefer a chunkier sauce, in step 2, instead of blending until smooth, pulse the ingredients 3 times or until your desired consistency is reached.

Serve over whole wheat pasta or try serving with spiralized zucchini noodles for a lighter meal.

• **Bullet blender with the extra-tall cup**

2 tbsp	sunflower oil	30 mL
½	onion, sliced and rings separated	½
2	cloves garlic, thinly sliced	2
6	plum (Roma) tomatoes, cored and quartered	6
1	chipotle chile pepper in adobo sauce (optional)	1
½	carrot, cut into chunks	½
2 tsp	granulated sugar	10 mL
¼ cup	lightly packed fresh basil leaves	60 mL
½ tsp	dried oregano	2 mL
½ tsp	lemon juice	2 mL
	Salt and freshly ground black pepper	

1. In a large saucepan, heat oil over medium-high heat until shimmering. Add onion and cook, stirring, for 6 minutes or until translucent. Add garlic and cook, stirring, for 1 minute or until fragrant. Add tomatoes, chipotle (if using) and carrot; cook, breaking up the tomatoes and stirring occasionally, for 7 to 9 minutes or until tomatoes are softened. Transfer to a large bowl and let cool.

2. Working in batches if necessary, add sugar, basil, oregano, lemon juice and cooled tomato mixture to the extra-tall cup. Twist the extractor blade onto the cup to seal. Blend for 30 seconds or until smooth.

3. Return sauce to the pan and cook over medium-low heat, stirring occasionally, for 5 minutes or until heated through. Season to taste with salt and pepper.

NUTRIENTS PER ½ CUP (125 ML)	
IF rating	65
Calories	70
Fat	5 g
Protein	1 g
Carbohydrate	7 g
Fiber	1 g
Sodium	24 mg
Calcium	18 mg

Jean's Tomato Basil Sauce

This is Jean's favorite all-purpose tomato sauce, as it mixes up quickly to serve over whole-grain pasta.

TIPS: If you're using this sauce to make homemade pizza, add 1 tsp (5 mL) dried oregano.

Leftover sauce can be stored in an airtight container in the refrigerator for up to 1 week.

- **Immersion blender**

1 tbsp	olive oil	15 mL
1	onion, chopped	1
2	cloves garlic, crushed	2
1	can (28 oz/796 mL) no-salt-added diced tomatoes	1
2 tbsp	basil pesto	30 mL

1. In a large saucepan, heat oil over medium-low heat. Add onion and cook, stirring, for 2 to 4 minutes or until starting to soften. Add garlic and cook, stirring, for 3 to 5 minutes or until onion and garlic are softened.

2. Stir in tomatoes and bring to a boil. Remove from heat and, using the immersion blender in the pan, purée sauce, leaving some tomato pieces intact. Stir in pesto.

NUTRIENTS PER SERVING	
IF rating	85
Calories	80
Fat	4 g
Protein	1 g
Carbohydrate	11 g
Fiber	3 g
Sodium	63 mg
Calcium	12 mg

Lemon Pesto Sauce

MAKES ABOUT
⅓ CUP (75 ML)

This sauce is a perfect example of Mediterranean eating. Keep a supply in the freezer so you always have it on hand.

TIPS: When fresh basil is not available, replace with 1 cup (250 mL) fresh parsley leaves and 2 tbsp (30 mL) dried basil.

Basil contributes to healthy eating because it is a flavor enhancer, which reduces the need for fat and salt.

- **Food processor or blender**

1 cup	packed fresh basil leaves (see tips)	250 mL
1	clove garlic	1
1 tbsp	olive oil	15 mL
1 tbsp	almonds or pine nuts	15 mL
4 tsp	lemon juice	20 mL
1 tsp	grated lemon zest	5 mL

1. In food processor, combine basil, garlic, oil, almonds, lemon juice and zest. Blend until coarsely chopped. Chill or freeze, as desired.

This recipe courtesy of dietitian Margaret Howard.

NUTRIENTS PER 1 TBSP (15 ML)	
IF rating	48
Calories	39
Fat	4 g
Protein	1 g
Carbohydrate	1 g
Fiber	0 g
Sodium	1 mg
Calcium	21 mg

Black and White Bean Salsa

Serve over salad as a side dish. Also great over grains such as couscous or brown rice. On non-vegetarian days, try this salsa with fish or chicken.

1 cup	rinsed drained canned black beans	250 mL
1 cup	rinsed drained canned navy beans	250 mL
1 cup	chopped plum (Roma) tomatoes	250 mL
½ cup	canned corn, drained	125 mL
⅓ cup	chopped fresh cilantro	75 mL
⅓ cup	chopped green onions	75 mL
⅓ cup	chopped red bell pepper	75 mL
2 tbsp	freshly squeezed lime juice	30 mL
1½ tbsp	olive oil	22 mL
1½ tsp	chili powder	7 mL
1 tsp	minced garlic	5 mL
	Freshly ground black pepper	

1. In a bowl, combine black beans, navy beans, tomatoes, corn, cilantro, green onions, red pepper, lime juice, oil, chili powder and garlic; mix well. Season to taste with pepper.

NUTRIENTS PER ½ CUP (125 ML)	
IF rating	49
Calories	134
Fat	4 g
Protein	6 g
Carbohydrate	20 g
Fiber	7 g
Sodium	49 mg
Calcium	42 mg

Quick Roasted Red Pepper Dip

Roasted red peppers are flavorful and offer key nutrients. No wonder they are a common ingredient in many recipes. You can roast them yourself and freeze them for later use or purchase them already prepared in a jar. Serve this dip with raw vegetables and whole-grain pita bread triangles or whole wheat crackers.

TIP: Red peppers are high in antioxidant vitamins, including beta-carotene and vitamin C, and they are also anti-inflammatory superstars! Although many people believe all vegetables in the nightshade family are inflammatory, this seems to be true only for a minority of people with arthritis who experience more joint pain after ingesting solanine, an ingredient in nightshades. Unless you are one of these people, you can eat red peppers with confidence, knowing that they are anti-inflammatory.

NUTRIENTS PER 2 TBSP (30 ML)	
IF rating	32
Calories	61
Fat	4 g
Protein	3 g
Carbohydrate	3 g
Fiber	1 g
Sodium	173 mg
Calcium	95 mg

- **Food processor or blender**

3	roasted red bell peppers, skins and seeds removed (see box)	3
¾ cup	feta cheese, drained and crumbled (about 6 oz/175 g)	175 mL
½ tsp	minced garlic	2 mL
¼ tsp	hot pepper flakes	1 mL

1. In food processor, purée peppers, feta cheese, garlic and hot pepper flakes. Chill before serving.

This recipe courtesy of dietitian Helen Haresign.

Roasting Peppers

Preheat barbecue grill (you can broil in the oven as well, but it's easier and less messy on the barbecue and you can enjoy the outdoors). Place several peppers on the grill and cook until the skins turn black. Keep turning the peppers until the skins are blistered and black. Place the roasted peppers in large stockpot with a lid. The steam will make them sweat, so the skin will be easier to peel off. Let peppers cool, then remove stems, seeds and skin.

Fiery Verde Dip

Verde *means "green,"
and this hot and spicy dip
featuring jalapeño peppers
is a fresh alternative to
commercially prepared
guacamole and bean dips.
It's low in fat and high in
fiber. It goes great with
whole-grain pita bread
triangles, baked tortilla
chips and raw veggies.*

TIPS: Cilantro — also known
as fresh coriander or Chinese
parsley — has a pungent flavor
that you either love or hate.
Don't confuse it with ground
coriander, which is completely
different.

This dip keeps in the refrigerator
for up to 5 days.

- **Food processor or blender**

1	can (14 to 19 oz/398 to 540 mL) cannellini (white kidney) beans, drained and rinsed	1
½ cup	loosely packed fresh cilantro	125 mL
¼ cup	freshly squeezed lemon or lime juice	60 mL
1 tbsp	olive oil	15 mL
1 tsp	minced garlic	5 mL
1 or 2	jalapeño peppers, seeded and cut into chunks	1 or 2

1. In food processor, combine beans, cilantro, lemon juice, oil, garlic and peppers; blend until smooth. Chill before serving.

*This recipe courtesy of dietitians
Pamela Piotrowski and Shannon Crocker.*

NUTRIENTS PER 2 TBSP (30 ML)	
IF rating	31
Calories	96
Fat	3 g
Protein	5 g
Carbohydrate	13 g
Fiber	3 g
Sodium	134 mg
Calcium	37 mg

Fazool

Fagioli *is the Italian word for "beans," but people from Naples pronounce it "fazool," like in the Dean Martin song "That's Amore": "When the stars make you drool, just like pasta fazool, that's amore." In this case, fazool is a bean spread rather than pasta with beans. It's great on whole-grain crackers or as a substitute for butter or margarine, to reduce the fat and increase the protein (and flavor).*

TIPS: The ginger, balsamic vinegar and hot pepper sauce in this recipe add loads of flavor without fat.

This tasty spread is a healthy alternative to higher-fat spreads.

• **Food processor**

1 cup	white beans	250 mL
1	medium onion, chopped	1
3 tbsp	chopped gingerroot	45 mL
¾ tsp	salt, divided	3 mL
3 tbsp	olive oil	45 mL
2 tbsp	balsamic vinegar	30 mL
¼ tsp	hot pepper sauce	1 mL
Pinch	black pepper	Pinch

1. Cover beans with water; let soak overnight. Drain and rinse.

2. In a large saucepan, combine beans, onion, ginger, ½ tsp (2 mL) salt and enough water to cover; bring to a boil. Reduce heat and simmer, uncovered, until beans are tender, 35 to 40 minutes. Drain well.

3. In food processor, purée beans with oil, vinegar, hot pepper sauce, pepper and the remaining salt. Chill.

This recipe courtesy of chef Hans Anderegg and dietitian Cheryl Turnbull-Bruce.

NUTRIENTS PER 2 TBSP (30 ML)	
IF rating	98
Calories	81
Fat	5 g
Protein	2 g
Carbohydrate	8 g
Fiber	2 g
Sodium	198 mg
Calcium	24 mg

Slow-Roasted Garlic

MAKES 30 CLOVES

If you like to have roasted garlic on hand to use as a condiment or in recipes, here is a very easy way to make it. The garlic cooks away in the slow cooker and you can forget about it while you do other things. Store for up to 2 days, tightly covered, in the refrigerator or frozen in small portions for up to 3 months.

TIP: Double or triple this recipe to suit your needs.

- **Small (about 2-quart) slow cooker**
- **Large sheet of parchment paper**

30	cloves peeled garlic (about 2 heads)	30
2 tbsp	olive oil	30 mL

1. Lay parchment on a flat work surface and mound garlic in the middle. Spoon olive oil over garlic. Lift 2 opposite sides of parchment to meet in the middle, then fold them over to form a seal. Continue folding until flush with garlic. Fold the remaining sides over to form a package. Place in slow cooker, seam side down. Cover and cook on High for 4 hours, until garlic is nicely caramelized.

Uses for Roasted Garlic

There are many different ways to use roasted garlic. It's an easy way to enhance the flavor of simple soups, gravy or vinaigrettes. Just whisk in the desired quantity. It also makes a delicious addition to mashed potatoes or a great topping for grilled vegetables. Spread it over whole-grain crostini and top with fresh low-fat goat cheese for a delicious hors d'oeuvre. Simplest of all, spread it on whole-grain crackers or bread.

NUTRIENTS PER 1 TBSP (15 ML)	
IF rating	213
Calories	33
Fat	2 g
Protein	1 g
Carbohydrate	3 g
Fiber	0 g
Sodium	1 mg
Calcium	15 mg

Carrot, Raspberry and Oatmeal Breakfast Smoothie

Why not start your day with a dose of vegetables, fruits, grains and protein and feel like you did your body a favor? Carrots contain a phytonutrient called falcarinol, which has been shown to have promising anticancer properties. In addition, this smoothie provides beta- and alpha-carotene, flavonoids and vitamin C, making it a great source of anticancer compounds.

VARIATION: Add 1 to 1½ tsp (5 to 7 mL) açaí powder after the oats.

- **Bullet blender with the tall cup**

1	carrot, cut into chunks	1
1	banana, halved	1
½	orange, peeled and seeded	½
½ cup	raspberries	125 mL
½ cup	plain yogurt	125 mL
¼ cup	large-flake (old-fashioned) rolled oats	60 mL
	Unsweetened almond milk	

1. Add carrot, banana, orange, raspberries, yogurt and oats to the tall cup. Add almond milk to the "Max Line." Twist the extractor blade onto the cup to seal. Blend for 30 seconds or until smooth.

NUTRIENTS PER SERVING	
IF rating	4
Calories	360
Fat	5 g
Protein	13 g
Carbohydrate	70 g
Fiber	12 g
Sodium	209 mg
Calcium	522 mg

Carrot, Mango, Citrus and Ginger Smoothie with Hemp Seeds

Loaded with fruits, vegetables, a bit of spice and everything nice, this smoothie delivers great things to your body. This smoothie benefits any health condition with underlying inflammation and supports overall health.

TIP: You can substitute a ¼-inch (0.5 cm) square piece of fresh turmeric for the ground turmeric.

VARIATION: Add 1 to 1½ tsp (5 to 7 mL) açaí powder after the hemp seeds.

- **Bullet blender with the tall cup**

1	small carrot, cut into chunks	1
1	orange, peeled and seeded	1
1	½-inch (1 cm) square piece gingerroot	1
½ cup	frozen mango chunks	125 mL
½ cup	frozen pineapple chunks	125 mL
1 tbsp	hemp seeds	15 mL
¾ tsp	ground turmeric	3 mL
1½ tbsp	lemon juice	22 mL
	Water	

1. Add carrot, orange, ginger, mango, pineapple, hemp seeds, turmeric and lemon juice to the tall cup. Add water to the "Max Line." Twist the extractor blade onto the cup to seal. Blend for 40 seconds or until smooth.

NUTRIENTS PER SERVING	
IF rating	435
Calories	248
Fat	5 g
Protein	7 g
Carbohydrate	49 g
Fiber	9 g
Sodium	50 mg
Calcium	108 mg

Turmeric Ginger Tea

If you're not all that familiar with fresh turmeric or ginger and are wondering how to get more of them in your diet, one super-simple way is to make a fresh turmeric ginger tea. It couldn't be easier.

TIP: It wasn't possible to calculate the IF for this recipe, as the turmeric and ginger are steeped and not consumed directly. On their own, the turmeric root and gingerroot each have an IF of +147.

- **Tea pot**

1	3-inch (7.5 cm) piece fresh turmeric root	1
1	3-inch (7.5 cm) piece gingerroot	1
4 cups	boiling water	1 L

1. Scrub turmeric and ginger under running water. Cut into thick slices and place in tea pot. Fill with boiling water and let steep for 8 for 10 minutes or until desired strength. Strain into tea cups.

NUTRIENTS PER SERVING	
IF rating	n/a
Calories	15
Fat	0 g
Protein	0 g
Carbohydrate	3 g
Fiber	0 g
Sodium	1 mg
Calcium	7 mg

pH Levels of Skin Care Products

pH of Moisturizers Commonly Available in the United States

PRODUCT NAME	PH LEVEL
Acid mantle	4.71 ± 0.01
Aquanil lotion	5.19 ± 0.04
Aquanil HC	6.35 ± 0.12
Aquaphor ointment	6.84 ± 0.20
Aveeno daily moisturizing lotion	5.62 ± 0.01
Aveeno advanced care moisturizing cream	6.35 ± 0.03
Aveeno positively radiant daily moisturizer	5.54 ± 0.04
Aveeno skin relief moisturizing lotion	4.88 ± 0.02
Aveeno skin relief moisturizing lotion with menthol	5.46 ± 0.02
CeraVe moisturizing cream	5.49 ± 0.02
CeraVe moisturizing lotion	5.68 ± 0.02
CeraVe facial moisturizing lotion PM	5.95 ± 0.01
Cetaphil moisturizing cream	4.71 ± 0.02
Cetaphil RestoraDerm skin restoring moisturizer	5.94 ± 0.02
Cetaphil daily advance ultrahydrating lotion	5.65 ± 0.01
Dove day lotion	6.47 ± 0.02
DML forte body moisturizing cream	5.94 ± 0.08
DML moisturizing lotion	6.55 ± 0.01
Epiceram	5.45 ± 0.01
Eucerin calming cream	5.41 ± 0.02
Eucerin menthol itch relief lotion	4.81 ± 0.03
Eucerin original dry skin therapy cream	8.01 ± 0.04
Eucerin original dry skin therapy lotion	5.97 ± 0.03
Eucerin intensive repair body cream	5.98 ± 0.03
Eucerin intensive repair body lotion	8.19 ± 0.03
Neosalus cream	7.40 ± 0.10
Theraplex emollient for severely dry skin	4.62 ± 0.18
Vanicream moisturizing skin cream	4.27 ± 0.05
Vanicream light moisturizing lotion	3.73 ± 0.03
Vaseline intensive rescue skin protectant body lotion	4.30 ± 0.02

Source: *Adapted from Ali et al., 2013. Available at www.medicaljournals.se/acta/content/?doi=10.2340/00015555-1531.*

pH of Cleansers Commonly Available in the United States

PRODUCT NAME	PH LEVEL
Aderm	6.44
Avecyde	3.61
Avène	6.94
Camay classic	10.38
Camay gala	10.36
Camay soft	10.26
Cetaphil	7.72
Dove white	7.53
Dove baby	7.00
Dove liquid	5.16
Dove pink	7.23
Johnson's baby	11.90
Johnson's baby oat	12.35
Nivea baby cream	12.35
Nivea bath care	12.21
Nivea bath care almond	12.22
Nivea bath care oat	12.30
Palmolive green	10.18
Palmolive white	10.23
Palmolive botanicals	10.38
Palmolive botanicals chamomile	10.13
Zest neutral	9.85
Zest citrus sport	9.75
Zest herbal	9.97
Zest aqua	9.89

Source: *Adapted from Ali et al., 2013. Available at www.medicaljournals.se/acta/content/?doi=10.2340/00015555-1531.*

pH of Moisturizers Commonly Available in Canada

PRODUCT NAME	PH LEVEL* (as per manufacturer)
Aveeno daily moisture lotion	4.1–6.5
Aveeno skin relief moisturizing lotion	4.2–6.3
Cetaphil RestoraDerm moisturizer	5.5–6.1
Curel itch defense	4.0–6.0
Gold Bond ultimate	4.0–7.0
Johnson baby lotion	Not provided
Johnson natural baby lotion	4.3–4.9
Lubriderm advanced moisture therapy daily	6.0–7.5
Lubriderm intense dry skin repair body lotion	Not provided
Lubriderm unscented lotion	Not provided
Neutrogena Norwegian lotion	7.0–8.0
St. Ives	Not provided
Vaseline	Not provided
Vaseline intensive care advanced repair	5.0–7.0

*The companies tend to list a range for pH values. Choose products as close to the pH of the acid mantle (4.71 ± 0.01) as possible.

Source: *Data gathered by calling company customer service lines on product packaging.*

pH of Cleansers Commonly Available in Canada*

PRODUCT NAME	PH LEVEL** (as per manufacturer)
Aveeno moisturizing bar for dry skin	Not provided
Aveeno skin relief body wash, fragrance-free	4.3–5.1
Cetaphil gentle cleansing bar	6.75–7.75
Cetaphil gentle skin cleanser	5.5–7.0
Dove deep moisture body wash	6.0–7.3
Dove white bar soap	6.8–7.9
Ivory clean bar soap	10.4
Lever 2000 bar soap	8.0

*Bar soaps tend to have a higher (more alkaline) pH.

**The companies tend to list a range for pH values. Choose products as close to the pH of the acid mantle (4.71 ± 0.01) as possible.

Source: *Data gathered by calling company customer service lines on product packaging.*

APPENDIX 2: BMI Table

‹ BODY WEIGHT (lbs) ›

‹ HEIGHT (inches) ›

BMI	NORMAL						OVERWEIGHT					OBESE										EXTREME OBESITY											
	19	20	21	22	23	24	25	26	27	28	29	30	31	32	33	34	35	36	37	38	39	40	41	42	43	44	45	46	47	48	49	50
58	91	96	100	105	110	115	119	124	129	134	138	143	148	153	158	162	167	172	177	181	186	191	196	201	205	210	215	220	224	229	234	239
59	94	99	104	109	114	119	124	128	133	138	143	148	153	158	163	168	173	178	183	188	193	198	203	208	212	217	222	227	232	237	242	247
60	97	102	107	112	118	123	128	133	138	143	148	153	158	163	168	174	179	184	189	194	199	204	209	215	220	225	230	235	240	245	250	255
61	100	106	111	116	122	127	132	137	143	148	153	158	164	169	174	180	185	190	195	201	206	211	217	222	227	232	238	243	248	254	259	264
62	104	109	115	120	126	131	136	142	147	153	158	164	169	175	180	186	191	196	202	207	213	218	224	229	235	240	246	251	256	262	267	273
63	107	113	118	124	130	135	141	146	152	158	163	169	175	180	186	191	197	203	208	214	220	225	231	237	242	248	254	259	265	270	278	282
64	110	116	122	128	134	140	145	151	157	163	169	174	180	186	192	197	204	209	215	221	227	232	238	244	250	256	262	267	273	279	285	291
65	114	120	126	132	138	144	150	156	162	168	174	180	186	192	198	204	210	216	222	228	234	240	246	252	258	264	270	276	282	288	294	300
66	118	124	130	136	142	148	155	161	167	173	179	186	192	198	204	210	216	223	229	235	241	247	253	260	266	272	278	284	291	297	303	309
67	121	127	134	140	146	153	159	166	172	178	185	191	198	204	211	217	223	230	236	242	249	255	261	268	274	280	287	293	299	306	312	319
68	125	131	138	144	151	158	164	171	177	184	190	197	203	210	216	223	230	236	243	249	256	262	269	276	282	289	295	302	308	315	322	328
69	128	135	142	149	155	162	169	176	182	189	196	203	209	216	223	230	236	243	250	257	263	270	277	284	291	297	304	311	318	324	331	338
70	132	139	146	153	160	167	174	181	188	195	202	209	216	222	229	236	243	250	257	264	271	278	285	292	299	306	313	320	327	334	341	348
71	136	143	150	157	165	172	179	186	193	200	208	215	222	229	236	243	250	257	265	272	279	286	293	301	308	315	322	329	336	343	351	358
72	140	147	154	162	169	177	184	191	199	206	213	221	228	235	242	250	258	265	272	279	287	294	302	309	316	324	331	338	346	353	361	368
73	144	151	159	166	174	182	189	197	204	212	219	227	235	242	250	257	265	272	280	288	295	302	310	318	325	333	340	348	355	363	371	378
74	148	155	163	171	179	186	194	202	210	218	225	233	241	249	256	264	272	280	287	295	303	311	319	326	334	342	350	358	365	373	381	389
75	152	160	168	176	184	192	200	208	216	224	232	240	248	256	264	272	279	287	295	303	311	319	327	335	343	351	359	367	375	383	391	399
76	156	164	172	180	189	197	205	213	221	230	238	246	254	263	271	279	287	295	304	312	320	328	336	344	353	361	369	377	385	394	402	410

APPENDIX 3

Supplement Descriptions, Claims and Evidence

Berberine

A chemical found in various roots and plants, including goldenseal.
Product: Tablets.
Lymphedema claims: Fat burning.
Evidence of effectiveness: No evidence of effectiveness in lymphedema.

Burdock Root

(*Arctium lappa*, *Arctium minus*, *Arctium tomentosum*)
A root.
Products: Tea, edible root.
Lymphedema claims: Diuretic, anti-inflammatory.
Evidence of effectiveness: No evidence of effectiveness in lymphedema.

Butcher's-Broom

(*Ruscus aculeatus*)
A small evergreen shrub also known as box holly, fragon, Jew's myrtle and sweet broom.
An ingredient in Cyclo 3 Fort.
Products: Liquid extract, capsules, tea.
Lymphedema claim: Used to treat symptoms of chronic venous insufficiency (pain, heaviness, leg edema, cramps, itching and swelling).
Evidence of effectiveness: Taking a product called Cyclo 3 Fort (150 mg hesperidin, 150 mg butcher's-broom and 100 mg ascorbic acid per capsule) three times per day for 90 days reduced swelling in the upper arm and forearm and improved mobility and heaviness compared to placebo in women after breast cancer surgery (Cluzan, 1996). Not possible to draw conclusions about the effectiveness of this class of compounds (benzopyrones) in the management of lymphedema from the available research trials (Badger, 2004). Cyclo 3 Fort rated as "possibly effective" by the Natural Medicines Database (2015).

Calendula

(*Calendula officinalis*)
A flower with edible petals, also called marigold and gold-bloom. An ingredient in Traumeel ointment.
Active ingredients: Coumarins esculetin, scopoletin.
Products: Essential oil extract, topical cream, mouthwash.
Lymphedema claims: Anti-inflammatory; stimulates drainage of lymph nodes, especially in the breast and pelvic areas.
Evidence of effectiveness: No evidence of effectiveness in lymphedema.

Cleavers

(*Galium aparine*)
A flowering plant also known as catchweed, goosegrass and stickyweed.
Active ingredient: Galiosin.
Products: Tincture, tea.
Lymphedema claims: Increases lymphatic drainage, breaks up lymphatic congestion, anti-inflammatory.
Evidence of effectiveness: There is insufficient research to support its use for any human condition (Scheepers, 2006). No evidence of effectiveness in lymphedema.

Coumarin

A chemical found in many plants, including tonka beans (*Coumarouna odorata*), sweet clover and cassia (cinnamon).
Products: IV, tablets, cream.
Lymphedema claims: Stimulation of lymphatic function, reduces edema, anti-inflammatory.
Evidence of effectiveness: Improvement in mild lymphedema when used in addition to physiotherapy (Pecking, 1990). Improvement in lymphedema in 76 patients in open-label study with coumarin plus ginkgo biloba plus Melilotus and manual lymphatic drainage (Vettorello, 1996). No improvement in arm lymphedema in women after 6 months of coumarin, and 6% of the women developed liver toxicity (Loprinzi, 1999). Although effective, it isn't universally recommended until patients have a genetic screen done to determine if they're susceptible to liver toxicity from coumarin (Farinola, 2005).

Devil's Claw

(*Harpagophytum procumbens*)
A flowering plant with a large main root and tuberous branches, also known as hook plant and wood spider.
Products: Tablets, capsules, extract.
Lymphedema claims: Anti-inflammatory, diuretic.
Evidence of effectiveness: No evidence of effectiveness in lymphedema.

Diosmin

A bioflavonoid found in citrus. An ingredient in Daflon.

Products: Tablets, powder.

Lymphedema claims: Treatment of venous ulcers, anti-inflammatory, improves lymphatic drainage.

Evidence of effectiveness: Ten women with upper arm lymphedema following breast cancer received Daflon 500 mg twice a day for 6 months in non-blinded pilot study. Lymphedema improved, but it is not clear if they also received physiotherapy for lymphedema in addition to the supplement (Pecking, 1995). Two tablets of Daflon 500 mg per day in double-blind study with arm lymphedema showed improvement in speed of lymphatic migration but not the total lymph volume in severe lymphedema. No improvement in mild lymphedema over 6 months (Pecking, 1997). Not possible to draw conclusions about the effectiveness of this class of compounds (benzopyrones) in the management of lymphedema from the available research trials (Badger, 2004). Ranked as "possibly ineffective" by the Natural Medicines Database (2018).

Enzymes

Enzymes from cow, pig or ox pancreas (pancreatin, trypsin, chymotrypsin); pineapple fruit and stem (bromelain); and papaya (papain). Ingredients in Wobenzym N.

Product: Tablets.

Lymphedema claims: Treats swelling and pain.

Evidence of effectiveness: Wobenzym N plus manual and machine lymphatic drainage improved lymphedema of the arm as well as pain compared with diuretics plus manual and machine lymphatic drainage (Korpan, 1996).

French Oak Wood

(*Quercus robur*)

Wood and bark from the French oak, also called the sessile oak. Ingredient in Robuvit.

Active ingredients: Roburins, grandinin.

Product: Capsules.

Lymphedema claims: Anti-inflammatory, reduces edema.

Evidence of effectiveness: In patients with primary lymphedema in the leg, 300 mg and 600 mg of Robuvit plus standard therapy for 8 weeks improved lymphedema more than standard therapy alone (Belcaro, 2015).

Ginkgo

(*Ginkgo biloba*)

A tree also known as Japanese silver apricot or kew tree. An ingredient in BN 165 (Ginkor Fort).

Product: Capsules.

Lymphedema claim: May improve peripheral vascular disease.

Evidence of effectiveness: Patients with upper arm lymphedema secondary to breast cancer treatment were given 2 capsules per day of Ginkor Fort (ginkgo biloba plus troxerutin plus heptaminol hydrochloride) and showed improvement in limb heaviness and lymphatic migration speed compared to placebo (Cluzan, 2004).

Gotu Kola

(*Centella asiatica*)

A creeping plant in the parsley family.

Products: Tablets, cream.

Lymphedema claim: Treats venous insufficiency.

Evidence of effectiveness: Deemed as "possibly effective" in the treatment of venous insufficiency by Natural Medicines Database (2017). No evidence of effectiveness in lymphedema.

Hesperidin

A bioflavonoid found in many plants, especially unripe citrus. An ingredient in Daflon 500 and Cyclo 3 Fort.

Products: Tablets, cream.

Lymphedema claims: Anti-lymphedema, treats varicose veins and venous stasis (clotting).

Evidence of effectiveness: The product Daflon 500 (see Diosmin, page 247) contains 50 mg hesperidin and 450 mg diosmin per tablet. Taking a product called Cyclo 3 Fort (150 mg hesperidin, 150 mg butcher's-broom and 100 mg ascorbic acid per capsule) three times per day for 90 days reduced swelling in the upper arm and forearm and improved mobility and heaviness compared to placebo in women after breast cancer surgery (Cluzan, 1996). Not possible to draw conclusions about the effectiveness of this class of compounds (benzopyrones) in the management of lymphedema from the available research trials (Badger, 2004). The Natural Medicines Database ranks it "insufficient reliable evidence to rate for lymphedema" (2018).

Homeopathy

A dilute mixture of herbs, used in Itires and Lymph Stim Liquescence.

Product: Homeopathic tincture.

Lymphedema claim: Improves flow of lymph.

Evidence of effectiveness: Homeopathy is based on the "law of similars." Given there is no active ingredient in homeopathic preparations, any results are thought to be due to placebo effect. Most studies show homeopathy is ineffective.

Horse Chestnut

(*Aesculus hippocastanum*)

A seed (bark and leaf are also used), also called buckeye. An ingredient in Venoruton, Paroven, Venostasin, Essaven gel and Somatoline.

Active ingredients: Oxerutins and escin.

Products: Extract, topical gel, capsules, IV.

Lymphedema claims: Anti-inflammatory, edema-preventing action (chronic venous insufficiency).

Evidence of effectiveness: Improvement in edema due to chronic venous insufficiency with Venoruton, Paroven, Venostasin, Essaven gel and horse chestnut extract (Wollina, 2006; Underland, 2012). The product Somatoline showed satisfactory results when given along with traditional lymphedema treatment (Dini, 1981). A Cochrane review pooling results from seven studies found that horse chestnut seed extract improved leg pain and limb volume caused by chronic venous insufficiency (Pittler, 2012). In a trial with women with arm lymphedema following cancer treatment, horse chestnut failed to show any significant improvement in lymphedema (Huston, 2018, personal correspondence, unpublished research).

Jersey Tea

(*Ceanothus americanus*, *Ceanothus intermedius*)

Also known as New Jersey tea and red root.

Products: Liquid tincture, capsules.

Lymphedema claims: Promotes lymph flow and production, diuretic.

Evidence of effectiveness: No evidence of effectiveness in lymphedema.

L-arginine

An amino acid — 2-amino-5-guanidinopentanoic acid — found in meat, poultry, fish and dairy.

Lymphedema claims: Converts to nitric oxide and is responsible for widening blood vessels (vasodilator) and will have the same effect on lymph vessels.

Evidence of effectiveness: Deemed to be "possibly effective for treatment of peripheral vascular disease" by the Natural Medicines Database (2018). No evidence of effectiveness in lymphedema.

Madder

(*Rubia tinctorum*, *Rubia cordifolia*)

A perennial weed also known as Indian madder and manjistha.

Products: Powder, tablets.

Lymphedema claims: Supports movement and flow of the lymphatic system, treats cellulitis.

Evidence of effectiveness: In a detailed summary of all the documented uses of madder, lymphedema is absent (Priya, 2014). Considered "likely unsafe" and a possible carcinogen by Natural Medicines Database (2016).

Marshmallow Root

(*Althaea officinalis*)

An herb also known as mortification root and sweet weed.

Lymphedema claim: Anti-inflammatory.

Evidence of effectiveness: No evidence of effectiveness in lymphedema.

N-acetyl Cysteine

Made from the amino acid L-cysteine.

Products: Tablets, puffer, cream, IV.

Lymphedema claims: Antioxidant, anti-inflammatory, breaks down fat.

Evidence of effectiveness: No evidence of effectiveness in lymphedema.

Parsley Root

(*Petroselinum crispum*)

An herb also known as common parsley and garden parsley. The oil, root, leaf and seed have all been used in herbal medicine.

Products: Capsules, tea.

Lymphedema claims: Anti-edema, anti-inflammatory.

Evidence of effectiveness: In some situations, parsley could make edema worse. No evidence of effectiveness in lymphedema.

Pine Bark

(*Pinus pinaster*)

The bark of the Maritime pine. An ingredient in Pycnogenol.

Products: Tablets, cream, oil.

Lymphedema claims: Reduces leg pain and heaviness, reduces fluid retention.

Evidence of effectiveness: The use of Pycnogenol before a long flight prevented ankle edema better than placebo in normal subjects (Cesarone, 2005). In a trial with women with arm lymphedema following cancer treatment, Pycnogenol failed to show any significant improvement in lymphedema (Huston, 2018, personal correspondence, unpublished research).

Reishi Mushrooms

(*Ganoderma lucidum*)

A fungus also known as red reishi and spirit plant.

Products: Powder, liquid extract.

Lymphedema claims: Anti-inflammatory, antihypertensive.

Evidence of effectiveness: No evidence of effectiveness in lymphedema.

Rutin

A pigment of the bioflavonoid family found in many plants, especially citrus, capers, olives and buckwheat. An ingredient in Wobenzym N.

Products: Tablets, cream.

Lymphedema claims: Reduces lymphedema, strengthens blood vessels, anti-inflammatory.

Evidence of effectiveness: Wobenzym N plus manual and machine lymphatic drainage improved lymphedema of the arm as well as pain compared to diuretics plus manual and machine lymphatic drainage (Korpan, 1996).

Selenium

A mineral (sodium selenite) found in soil, water and food. An ingredient in Selenase.

Products: Tablets, IV, drinking ampules.

Lymphedema claims: Antioxidant, anti-edema.

Evidence of effectiveness: Selenium may help reduce the risk of bacterial skin infection (erysipelas) in women with lymphedema after breast cancer surgery (Kasseroller, 1998). Women with arm lymphedema post-mastectomy for cancer who received Selenase for 28 days had less lymphedema, better response to physical decongestion therapy, improved mobility and heat tolerance compared with placebo controls (Kasseroller, 2000). Forty-eight patients who had radiation- or surgery-plus-radiation-induced lymphedema of the arm (12) or head and neck (36) completed a trial of sodium selenite in the form of Selenase ampules for 4 to 6 weeks. The patients completed self-assessment before and after the supplementation, which indicated that they perceived their lymphedema had lessoned following the selenium (Micke, 2003). In a similar trial, sodium selenite in the form of Selenase was given for 4 to 6 weeks to 36 head-and-neck cancer patients. A majority experienced an improvement in their lymphedema and quality of life (Bruns, 2004). Three doses of 1,000 µg of sodium selenite IV before the day of oral cancer surgery and on the day of oral cancer surgery, plus 1000 µg oral or IV for 21 days post-surgery, significantly reduced lymphedema compared to placebo (Zimmermann, 2005). A Cochrane review of selenium in cancer side effects concluded that research to date does not provide evidence in favor of or against selenium supplementation for cancer side effects including secondary lymphedema (Dennert, 2006). Blood selenium levels were found to be lowest in the more severe (Stage 3) versus mildest (Stage 1) lymphedema and in morbidly obese individuals, and blood selenium levels were found to be higher in primary versus secondary lymphedema. This suggests that there may be increased selenium requirements in more severe cases of lymphedema, especially secondary lymphedema that is accompanied by morbid obesity (Pfister, 2016).

Turmeric

(*Curcuma longa*)

A root.

Active ingredient: Curcumin.

Products: Tablets, cream, enema.

Lymphedema claim: Anti-inflammatory.

Evidence of effectiveness: No evidence of effectiveness in lymphedema.

Vitamin E

(Alpha-tocopherol)

A fat-soluble vitamin found in many foods.

Product: Tablets.

Evidence of effectiveness: Vitamin E plus pentoxifylline in patients with arm lymphedema after surgery and radiation for breast cancer failed to improve lymphedema after 12 months versus placebo (Gothard, 2004).

Glossary

acute kidney disease: A sudden onset of kidney damage with a buildup of waste in the blood.

aortic aneurysm: An enlargement of the aorta, which is a blood vessel attached to the heart.

arm lymphedema: A 10% increase of swelling in the affected arm compared to the unaffected arm and lasting for 6 months or more.

axilla: The armpit area.

axillary lymph node dissection: Also called ALND, axillary dissection, axillary node dissection or axillary lymphadenectomy. Between one and 40 lymph nodes are removed from the armpit, based on the surgeon's judgment during the operation. The removed nodes are examined by a pathologist to determine if they contain cancer.

B cells: Also known a B lymphocytes, a type of white blood cell. They mature in the bone marrow (hence the *B*) and are part of the immunity you acquire when you are exposed to different antigens.

bile: A chemical made in the liver and stored in the gallbladder. It is released into the intestines from the common bile duct and helps the body digest oil and fat from the diet (also called gall).

body mass index (BMI): A mathematical calculation based on your height and weight to determine your risk of health problems related to weight (over and under). See also Appendix 2: BMI Table.

botanicals: Substances and medicines derived from plants.

bronchial asthma: An inflammatory condition of the breathing tubes of the lungs, making breathing difficult. The presence of bronchial asthma is an important consideration before performing MLD.

carcinoma: Cancer in the epithelial cells. This includes cancer of the prostate, bladder, lung, breast, ovaries, cervix, head and neck.

cardiovascular disease: Disease of the heart or blood vessels.

case study: A description of a single or small number of subjects and their experience with a particular condition or intervention.

chyle: Lymphatic fluid that is milky from emulsified fats (cholesterol, phospholipids, triglycerides and apolipoproteins). It is transported by the lacteals, specialized lymphatic capillaries that absorb dietary fats in the small intestine.

chylomicron: A small milky lipoprotein that contains triglycerides and other particles that allow for the transportation of fats from the intestines to other parts of the body.

chyme: A pulpy, acidic mixture of stomach acid and partially digested food that passes from the stomach to the small intestine.

clinical trial: Testing one treatment against a standard using human subjects. For example, testing a new bandage compared to a standard bandage.

colitis: Inflammation of the inner lining of the colon.

collagen: The main structural protein in the spaces between cells in connective tissue.

congestive heart failure: Heart failure with a buildup of fluid around the heart and edema in the ankles, feet and legs.

Crohn's disease: Inflammation of the bowel, which leads to inflammation of the digestive tract. It causes abdominal pain, diarrhea, weight loss and malnutrition.

deep vein thrombosis (DVT): Also called acute DVT or venous thrombosis, this is a blood clot (thrombus) that forms in a deep vein in the body. It can cause pain and swelling or no symptoms at all.

diverticulosis: In this intestinal disorder, pouches form in the walls of the colon.

early intervention: Identifying and providing effective treatment early.

epithelial cell: One of the four basic cell types that makes up tissue in the human body. These cells line the organs and blood vessels.

essential fatty acids: Fat is made up of fatty acids. Most fatty acids can be made by the body. The two that can't be made are called linoleic acid and alpha-linolenic acid. These essential fatty acids must be consumed in the diet.

fatty acids: As part of digestion, fats and oils are broken down into fatty acids. They can be classified by length as short-, medium- or long-chain.

fibrosis: The thickening of connective tissue.

gastrointestinal (GI): Relating to the stomach and intestines ("gastro" refers to the stomach, and "intestinal" to the small and large intestines).

gastrointestinal tract: This digestive path includes the entire length of the GI system, from the mouth to the anus.

genetic link: A problem caused by one or more abnormalities in the genome is passed down from one generation to the next.

gut-associated lymphatic tissue (GALT): The tissue that makes up the lining of the intestines, the largest amount of lymphoid tissue in the body.

hypertension: High blood pressure.

hyperthyroidism: An overactive thyroid gland releases an excess of the hormone thyroxine.

incidence rate: The rate of occurrence of a new diagnosis during a period of time.

inflammation: This can be acute (short-term) or chronic (long-term). The acute phase is a normal healthy response to an injury or to foreign cells. It is characterized by heat, pain, swelling, redness and loss of function. Acute inflammation resolves and the area goes back to normal. Chronic inflammation begins with the same response but the area doesn't return to normal and the environment can allow new disease to flourish, such as cancer and heart disease.

interstitial fluid: The fluid in the spaces between cells.

intravenous (IV): Administered into a vein.

ischemic vascular disease (IVD): A waxy substance called plaque builds up on the inside of the blood vessels and restricts the flow of blood.

lacteal: A lymphatic capillary of the small intestine that absorbs fat.

lipase: An enzyme that breaks down fat in the digestive tract. These have different names depending on their location — for example, salivary lipase (in the saliva of the mouth), gastric lipase (in the stomach) and pancreatic lipase (in the pancreas).

longitudinal study: A research study that gathers information on the same study subjects repeatedly over many years.

lymph: Fluid that enters the lymphatic system is initially very similar to blood plasma (clear or slightly milky in appearance). It contains water, protein, dead cells, bacteria and viruses. As it moves from lymph capillaries to larger lymph vessels, it's mixed with more protein, long-chain fatty acids, white blood cells and cellular debris, and it becomes more milky in appearance.

lymphadenectomy: The surgical removal of lymph nodes.

lymphangiogenesis: The genesis (creation) of new lymphatic vessels.

lymphatic vessel: Thin vessels throughout the body that carry lymph fluid.

lymphedema: A chronic condition caused by abnormal development of the lymphatic vessels or nodes (primary lymphedema) or from damage to the lymphatic vessels (secondary lymphedema). Also spelled lymphoedema.

macrophages: White blood cells that are an important part of the immune system. They engulf and consume foreign cells.

MCT oil: Medium-chain triglyceride oil is made from coconut and/or palm kernel oil and contains only fatty acids that are 6 to 12 carbons in length.

metabolism: Often described as the "body's engine," this involves the chemical processes that allow the body to perform normal functions, including converting food to energy.

metastasis: Cancer that has spread to a new area of the body.

near-infrared imaging: A sophisticated tool that scientists use to visualize objects that are impossible to see with the naked eye — for example, lymph capillaries.

nutrition: The science that studies how food and the body work together for health.

obesity: The excessive storage of fat in the body, or a BMI of 30 or higher.

peripheral neuropathy: Nerve damage affecting the hands and feet, which can result in weakness, pain and numbness.

peristalsis: The contraction and relaxation of muscles that moves food through the GI tract. Peristalsis is also used to circulate lymph in the lymph capillaries.

physiology: A science that studies how the body functions.

portal circulation: Blood passes from the gastrointestinal tract, pancreas and spleen through the portal vein to the liver.

portal vein: A short, thick vein with smaller collecting veins from the GI tract, gallbladder, pancreas and spleen; it takes blood to the liver.

pulmonary embolism: A blood clot that forms in one of the arteries leading from the heart to the lungs.

randomized control trial: A type of scientific experiment that randomly divides a larger group into two or more smaller groups — one or more of the groups receives a treatment and one (the control group) does not (no treatment or standard treatment).

renal failure: A gradual loss of kidney function in which waste products accumulate in the blood.

repetitive limb movements: Repeating the same movement over and over again, as is required by certain jobs or hobbies (such as stacking shelves or rowing a boat).

research: The scientific investigation into a particular topic.

resistance exercise: Any exercise that forces muscles to contract against an external weight.

sentinel lymph node dissection: Also called SLND, this is the removal of the first lymph node or nodes closest to a cancer tumor. The removed nodes are examined by a pathologist to determine if they contain cancer.

skin thickness: Human skin thickness varies from 0.02 inch (0.5 mm) thick on the eyelids to 0.16 inch (4 mm) on the heels of your feet. Lymphedema can cause a thickening of the skin and is often measured in research studies as a reflection of the health of the skin.

supplement: A vitamin, mineral or herbal product that is taken in pill or capsule form. It is not considered a pharmaceutical and therefore is not well regulated.

T cells: Also known as T lymphocytes, a type of white blood cell. These mature in the thymus (hence the *T*) and are part of the immunity you acquire when you are exposed to different antigens.

thrombus: A blood clot.

triglycerides: The main component of body fat for humans and other animals, and the main ingredient in vegetable oil. They are three to four fatty acids held together with glycerol.

vicious cycle: Also known as a vicious circle, this is a repeating cycle of one problem causing another problem, making the first problem worse.

Waldmann's disease: Also called primary intestinal lymphangiectasia (PIL), this is a rare disease characterized by enlarged lymph vessels leading to the small intestine. It is managed with a low-fat diet plus MCT oil.

Resources

Here are some online resources you can access for more information about lymphedema, bandaging supplies, training schools, nutrition support and herbal products. In addition to the sources below, you may also access online and in-person support groups in your area.

Lymphedema Associations, Organizations and Resources

United States

Lymphedema Treatment Act: https://lymphedematreatmentact.org/resources
Lymphatic Education & Research Network: https://lymphaticnetwork.org
Lymphedema Guru Blog: www.lymphedemablog.com
National Lymphedema Network: https://lymphnet.org

Canada

Canadian Lymphedema Framework: https://canadalymph.ca
Alberta Lymphedema Association: www.albertalymphedema.com
Atlantic Clinical Lymphedema Network: www.atlanticlymph.ca
British Columbia Lymphedema Association: www.bclymph.org
Lymphedema Association of Manitoba: www.lymphmanitoba.ca
Lymphedema Association of Newfoundland and Labrador: www.lymphnl.com
Lymphedema Association of Nova Scotia: https://lymphedemanovascotia.com
Lymphedema Association of Ontario: www.lymphontario.ca
Lymphedema Association of Quebec: www.infolympho.ca
Lymphedema Association of Saskatchewan: www.sasklymph.ca

North America

Lymphology Association of North America (LANA): www.clt-lana.org

United Kingdom

British Lymphology Society: www.thebls.com
Lymphoedema Support Network: www.lymphoedema.org

Australasia

Australasian Lymphology Association: www.lymphoedema.org.au

International

International Lymphoedema Framework: www.lympho.org

Cancer and Lymphedema

American Cancer Society: www.cancer.org/treatment/treatments-and-side-effects/
physical-side-effects/lymphedema/what-is-lymphedema.html

Canadian Cancer Society: www.cancer.ca/en/cancer-information/diagnosis-and-treatment/
managing-side-effects/lymphedema/?region=on

National Institutes of Health: www.cancer.gov/about-cancer/treatment/side-effects/
lymphedema/lymphedema-hp-pdq

Bandaging Supplies

Academy Bandages: http://lymphedemastore.com

Bandages Plus: www.bandagesplus.com

BrightLife Direct: www.brightlifedirect.com/collections/bandages

Canadian Bandage Shoppe: www.cdnbandageshop.com

Linotrade: www.lympholino.com

Lymphedema Products: www.lymphedemaproducts.com/products/lymphedema-
bandaging-kits.html

Performance Health: www.performancehealth.com/patient-arm-bandaging-kit

Training Schools

Academy of Lymphatic Studies: www.acols.com

Casley-Smith International: www.casleysmithinternational.org

Dr. Vodder School International: www.vodderschool.com

International Lymphedema and Wound Training Institute: www.ilwti.com

Klose Training & Consulting: www.klosetraining.com

LymphEd: www.lymphed.com

National Lymphedema Network: www.lymphnet.org

Norton School of Lymphatic Therapy: www.nortonschool.com

Integrated Lymph Drainage: www.torontolymphocare.com

Nutrition Support

United States: EatRight, Academy of Nutrition and Dietetics, www.eatright.org

Canada: Dietitians of Canada, www.dietitians.ca

United Kingdom: Association of U.K. Dietitians, www.bda.uk.com

Herbal Products

Health Canada Natural Health Products Database: https://health-products.canada.ca/
lnhpd-bdpsnh/index-eng.jsp

Mayo Clinic: www.mayoclinic.org

Memorial Sloan Kettering Cancer Center: www.mskcc.org

National Institutes of Health, Office of Dietary Supplements: https://ods.od.nih.gov

Natural Medicines Comprehensive Database: http://naturaldatabaseconsumer.
therapeuticresearch.com/home.aspx?cs=&s=NDC (an excellent resource but
requires a subscription)

References

Sources Used Throughout

Földi M, Földi E. *Földi's Textbook of Lymphology*. Munich, Germany: Urban & Fischer, 2012.

Thibodeau GA, Patton, KT. *Anatomy & Physiology*. St. Louis, MO: Mosby Elsevier, 2007.

Zuther JE, Norton S. *Lymphedema Management: The Comprehensive Guide for Practitioners, 3rd Edition*. Stuttgart, New York: Thieme Publishers, 2012.

Preface

PDQ Supportive and Palliative Care Editorial Board. PDQ lymphedema. *National Cancer Institute*. Updated Jul 17, 2015. Available at: www.cancer.gov/about-cancer/treatment/side-effects/lymphedema/lymphedema-hp-pdq. Accessed Mar 17, 2019.

Chapter 1: The Lymphatic System and Lymphedema

Alexander JS, Ganta VC, Jordan PA, et al. Gastrointestinal lymphatics in health and disease. *Pathophysiology*. 2010 Sep; 17 (4): 315–35.

Archambeau JO, Pezner R, Wasserman T. Pathophysiology of irradiated skin and breast. *Int J Radiat Oncol Biol Phys*. 1995 Mar 30; 31 (5): 1171–85.

Burt J, White G. *Lymphedema: A Breast Cancer Patient's Guide to Prevention and Healing*. Alameda, CA: Hunter House, 1999.

Casley-Smith JR, Morgan RG, Piller NB. Treatment of lymphedema of the arms and legs with 5,6-benzo-[α]-pyrone. *N Engl J Med*. 1993 Oct 14; 329 (16): 1158–63.

Deng J, Ridner SH, Dietrich MS, et al. Prevalence of secondary lymphedema in patients with head and neck cancer. *J Pain Symptom Manage*. 2012 Feb; 43 (2): 244–52.

Executive Committee. The diagnosis and treatment of peripheral lymphedema: 2016 consensus document of the International Society of Lymphology. *Lymphology*. 2016 Dec; 49 (4): 170–84.

Keast D, Towers A. The rising prevalence of lymphedema in Canada: A continuing dialogue. *Pathways*. Spring 2017: 5–8.

Lawanda BD, Mondry TE, Johnstone PA. Lymphedema: A primer on the identification and management of a chronic condition in oncologic treatment. *CA Cancer J Clin*. 2009 Jan–Feb; 59 (1): 8–24.

Liao SF, Li SH, Huang HY, et al. The efficacy of complex decongestive physiotherapy (CDP) and predictive factors of lymphedema severity and response to CDP in breast cancer-related lymphedema (BCRL). *Breast*. 2013 Oct; 22 (5): 703–6.

Lymphoedema Framework. Best practice for the management of lymphoedema. International consensus. London: MEP Ltd, 2006. *International Consensus*. 2006. Available at: www.lympho.org/wp-content/uploads/2016/03/Best_practice.pdf. Accessed Mar 17, 2019.

NLN Medical Advisory Committee. Position statement of National Lymphedema Network: The diagnosis and treatment of lymphedema. *National Lymphedema Network*. Feb 2011. Available at: https://issuu.com/lymphnet/docs/pp_2011_-_diagnosis.treatment. Accessed Jan 3, 2011.

NLN Medical Advisory Committee. Position statement of National Lymphedema Network: Training of lymphedema therapists. *National Lymphedema Network*. May 2010. Available at: https://issuu.com/lymphnet/docs/pp_2010_trainingtherapists. Accessed Mar 17, 2019.

Ogawa Y. Recent advances in medical treatment for lymphoedema. *Ann Vasc Dis*. 2012; 5 (2): 139–44.

Shaitelman SF, Cromwell KD, Rasmussen JC, et al. Recent progress in the treatment and prevention of cancer-related lymphedema. *CA Cancer J Clin*. 2015 Jan–Feb; 65 (1): 55–81.

Sompayrac L. *How the Immune System Works*. Hoboken, NJ: Wiley-Blackwell, 2012.

Chapter 2: Lymphedema Risk Reduction

Asdourian MS, Skolny MN, Brunelle C, et al. Precautions for breast cancer-related lymphoedema: Risk from air travel, ipsilateral arm blood pressure measurements, skin puncture, extreme temperatures, and cellulitis. *Lancet Oncol*. 2016 Sep; 17 (9): e392–405.

Bernas M. Assessment and risk reduction in lymphedema. *Semin Oncol Nurs*. 2013 Feb; 29 (1): 12–9.

Box RC, Reul-Hirche HM, Bullock-Saxton JE, et al. Physiotherapy after breast cancer surgery: Results of a randomised controlled study to minimise lymphoedema. *Breast Cancer Res Treat*. 2002 Sep; 75 (1): 51–64.

Casley-Smith JR, Casley-Smith JR. Lymphedema initiated by aircraft flights. *Aviat Space Environ Med*. 1996 Jan; 67 (1): 52–6.

Fu RM. Breast cancer-related lymphedema: Symptoms, diagnosis, risk reduction, and management. *World J Clin Oncol*. 2014 Aug 10; 5 (3): 241–7.

Greene AK, Grant FD, Slavin SA. Lower-extremity lymphedema and elevated body-mass index. *N Engl J Med*. 2012 May 31; 366 (22): 2136–7.

Hayes S, Cornish B, Newman B. Comparison of methods to diagnose lymphedema among breast cancer survivors: 6-month follow-up. *Breast Cancer Res Treat*. 2005 Feb; 89 (3): 221–6.

Mehrara BJ, Greene AK. Lymphedema and obesity: Is there a link? *Plast Reconstr Surg*. 2014 Jul; 134 (1): 154e–160e.

Rebegea L, Firescu D, Dumitru M, et al. The incidence and risk factors for occurrence of arm lymphedema after treatment of breast cancer. *Chirurgia (Bucur)*. 2015 Jan–Feb; 110 (1): 33–7.

Ridner SH, Dietrich MS, Stewart BR, et al. Body mass index and breast cancer treatment-related lymphedema. *Support Care Cancer*. 2011 Jun; 19 (6): 853–7.

Stout Gergich NL, Pfalzer LA, McGarvey C, et al. Preoperative assessment enables the early diagnosis and successful treatment of lymphedema. *Cancer*. 2008 Jun 15; 112 (12): 2809–19.

Chapter 3: Skin Care

Ali SM, Yosipovitch G. Skin pH: From basic science to basic skin care. *Acta Derm Venereol*. 2013 May; 93 (3): 261–7.

Al-Niaimi F, Cox N. Cellulitis and lymphedema: A vicious cycle. *J Lymphedema*. 2009; 4 (2): 38–42.

Fife CE, Farrow W, Hebert AA, et al. Skin and wound care in lymphedema patients: A taxonomy, primer, and literature review. *Adv Skin Wound Care*. 2017 Jul; 30 (7): 305–18.

Flour M. Dermatological issues in lymphoedema and chronic oedema. *J Com Nurs*. 2013; 27 (2): 27–32.

Joseph A, Mony P, Prasad M, et al. The efficacies of affected-limb care with penicillin, diethylcarbamazine, the combination of both drugs or antibiotic ointment, in the prevention of acute adenolymphangitis during bancroftian filariasis. *Ann Trop Med Parasitol*. 2004 Oct; 98 (7): 685–96.

Rawlings AV, Davies A, Carlomusto M, et al. Effect of lactic acid isomers on keratinocyte ceramide synthesis, stratum corneum lipid levels and stratum corneum barrier function. *Arch Dermatol Res.* 1996 Jun; 288 (7): 383–90.

Yosipovitch G, Maibach HI. Skin surface pH: A protective acid mantle. *Cosmet Toiletries.* 1996; 111: 101–2.

Chapter 4: Manual Lymphatic Drainage

Douglass J, Graves P, Gordon S. Self-care for management of secondary lymphedema: A systematic review. *PLoS Negl Trop Dis.* 2016 Jun 8; 10 (6): e0004740.

Földi E. The treatment of lymphedema. *Cancer.* 1998 Dec 15; 83 (12 Suppl American): 2833–4.

Hutzschenreuter P, Brümmer H, Ebberfeld K. Experimental and clinical studies of the mechanism of effect of manual lymph drainage therapy. [Article in German.] *Z Lymphol.* 1989 Jul; 13 (1): 62–4.

Karhail SK, Kaur M, Sambyal S, et al. Effect of manual lymphatic drainage in comparison to resistance training on lymphedema in post-surgical breast cancer patients. *Physiotherapy.* 2015; 101 (1): 722–3.

Langfield S, McFarland J. *Where the Rivers Meet the Sea: Using the Body Mind Spirit Connections in the Management of Lymphedema.* Cookstown Centre for Wellness: Self-published, 2009.

Leduc O, Bourgeois P, Leduc A. Manual lymphatic drainage: Scintigraphic demonstration of its efficacy on colloidal protein reabsorption. *Progress in Lymphology.* 1988; 551–4.

McNeely ML, Magee DL, Lees AW, et al. The addition of manual lymph drainage to compression therapy for breast cancer related lymphedema: A randomized controlled trial. *Breast Cancer Res Treat.* 2004 Jul; 86 (2): 95–106.

Shao Y, Zhong DS. Manual lymphatic drainage for breast cancer-related lymphedema. *Eur J Cancer Care (Engl).* 2017 Sep; 26 (5).

Williams AF, Vadgama A, Franks PJ, et al. A randomized controlled crossover study of manual lymphatic drainage therapy in women with breast cancer-related lymphoedema. *Eur J Cancer Care (Engl).* 2002 Dec; 11 (4): 254–61.

Zuther JE, Norton S. *Lymphedema Management: The Comprehensive Guide for Practitioners, 3rd Edition.* Stuttgart, New York: Thieme Publishers, 2012.

Chapter 5: Multilayer Compression Bandaging

Badger CM, Peacock JL, Mortimer PS. A randomized, controlled, parallel-group clinical trial comparing multilayer bandaging followed by hosiery versus hosiery alone in the treatment of patients with lymphedema of the limb. *Cancer.* 2000 Jun 15; 88 (12): 2832–7.

International Lymphoedema Framework. Compression therapy: A position document on compression bandaging. *International Lymphoedema Framework.* Jun 2012. Available at: www.lympho.org/wp-content/uploads/2016/03/Compression-bandaging-final.pdf. Accessed Mar 17, 2019.

Johansson K, Albertsson M, Ingvar C, et al. Effects of compression bandaging with or without manual lymph drainage treatment in patients with postoperative arm lymphedema. *Lymphology.* 1999 Sep; 32 (3): 103–10.

King M, Deveaux A, White H, et al. Compression garments versus compression bandaging in decongestive lymphatic therapy for breast cancer-related lymphedema: A randomized controlled trial. *Support Care Cancer.* 2012 May; 20 (5): 1031–6.

Chapter 6: Compression Garments

Boris M, Weindorf S, Lasinski BB. The risk of genital edema after external pump compression for lower limb lymphedema. *Lymphology*. 1998 Mar; 31 (1): 15–20.

Hansdorfer-Korzon R, Teodorczyk J, Gruszecka A, et al. Are compression corsets beneficial for the treatment of breast cancer-related lymphedema? New opportunities in physiotherapy treatment — a preliminary report. *Onco Targets Ther*. 2016 Apr 7; 9: 2089–98.

International Lymphoedema Framework. Compression therapy: A position document on compression bandaging. *International Lymphoedema Framework*. Jun 2012. Available at: www.lympho.org/wp-content/uploads/2016/03/Compression-bandaging-final.pdf. Accessed Mar 17, 2019.

Lymphedema Framework. *Template for Practice: Compression Hosiery in Lymphedema*. London: MEP Ltd, 2006.

Lymphoedema Framework. Best practice for the management of lymphoedema: International consensus. London: MEP Ltd, 2006. *International Consensus*. 2006. Available at: www.lympho.org/wp-content/uploads/2016/03/Best_practice.pdf. Accessed Mar 17, 2019.

Chapter 7: Pneumatic Compression Pumps

Boris M, Weindorf S, Lasinski BB. The risk of genital edema after external pump compression for lower limb lymphedema. *Lymphology*. 1998 Mar; 31 (1): 15–20.

Lymphoedema Framework. Best practice for the management of lymphoedema: International consensus. London: MEP Ltd, 2006. *International Consensus*. 2006. Available at: www.lympho.org/wp-content/uploads/2016/03/Best_practice.pdf. Accessed Mar 17, 2019.

Miranda F Jr, Perez MC, Castiglioni ML, et al. Effect of sequential intermittent pneumatic compression on both leg lymphedema volume and on lymph transport as semi-quantitatively evaluated by lymphoscintigraphy. *Lymphology*. 2001 Sep; 34 (3): 135–41.

NLN Medical Advisory Committee. Position statement of National Lymphedema Network: The diagnosis and treatment of lymphedema. *National Lymphedema Network*. Feb 2011. Available at: https://issuu.com/lymphnet/docs/pp_2011_-_diagnosis.treatment. Accessed Jan 3, 2011.

Shao Y, Qi K, Zhou QH, et al. Intermittent pneumatic compression pump for breast cancer-related lymphedema: A systematic review and meta-analysis of randomized controlled trials. *Oncol Res Treat*. 2014; 37 (4): 170–4.

Zuther JE, Norton S. *Lymphedema Management: The Comprehensive Guide for Practitioners, 3rd Edition*. Stuttgart, New York: Thieme Publishers, 2012.

Chapter 8: Exercise and Lymphedema

Baumann FT, Reike A, Reimer V, et al. Effects of physical exercise on breast cancer-related secondary lymphedema: A systematic review. *Breast Cancer Res Treat*. 2018 Jul; 170 (1): 1–13.

Brorson H, Ohlin K, Olsson G, et al. Adipose tissue dominates chronic arm lymphedema following breast cancer: An analysis using volume rendered CT images. *Lymphat Res Biol*. 2006; 4 (4): 199–210.

Brorson H, Ohlin K, Olsson G, et al. Quality of life following liposuction and conservative treatment of arm lymphedema. *Lymphology*. 2006 Mar; 39 (1): 8–25.

DiBlasio A, Morano T, Bucci I, et al. Physical exercises for breast cancer survivors: Effects of 10 weeks of training on upper limb circumferences. *J Phys Ther Sci*. 2016 Oct; 28 (10): 2778–84.

Di Blasio A, Morano T, Napolitano G, et al. Nordic walking and the Isa method for breast cancer survivors: Effects on upper limb circumferences and total body extracellular water — a pilot study. *Breast Care (Basel)*. 2016 Dec; 11 (6): 428–31.

Douglass J, Immink M, Piller N, et al. Yoga for women with breast cancer-related lymphoedema: A preliminary 6-month study. *J Lymphoedema*. 2012 Dec; 7 (2): 30–8.

Földi M, Földi E. *Földi's Textbook of Lymphology*. Munich, Germany: Urban & Fischer, 2012.

Fukushima T, Tsuji T, Sano Y, et al. Immediate effects of active exercise with compression therapy on lower-limb lymphedema. *Support Care Cancer*. 2017 Aug; 25 (8): 2603–10.

Galantino ML, Stout NL. Exercise interventions for upper limb dysfunction due to breast cancer treatment. *Phys Ther*. 2013 Oct; 93 (10): 1291–7.

Johansson K, Hayes S, Speck RM, et al. Water-based exercise for patients with chronic arm lymphedema: A randomized controlled pilot trial. *Am J Phys Med Rehabil*. 2013 Apr; 92 (4): 312–9.

Jönsson C, Johansson K. The effects of pole walking on arm lymphedema and cardiovascular fitness in women treated for breast cancer: A pilot and feasibility study. *Physiother Theory Pract*. 2014 May; 30 (4): 236–42.

Katz E, Dugan NL, Cohn JC, et al. Weight lifting in patients with lower-extremity lymphedema secondary to cancer: A pilot and feasibility study. *Arch Phys Med Rehabil*. 2010 Jul; 91 (7): 1070–6.

Loudon A, Barnett T, Piller N, et al. Yoga management of breast cancer-related lymphoedema: A randomised controlled pilot-trial. *BMC Complement Altern Med*. 2014 Jul 1; 14: 214.

Malicka I, Stefanska M, Rudziak M, et al. The influence of Nordic walking exercise on upper extremity strength and the volume of lymphoedema in women following breast cancer treatment. *Isokinetics Exerc Sci*. 2011; 19: 295–304.

Moadel AB, Shah C, Wylie-Rosett J, et al. Randomized controlled trial of yoga among a multiethnic sample of breast cancer patients: Effects on quality of life. *J Clin Oncol*. 2007 Oct 1; 25 (28): 4387–95.

NLN Medical Advisory Committee. Position statement of National Lymphedema Network: Exercise. *National Lymphedema Network*. Dec 2011. Available at: https://issuu.com/lymphnet/docs/exercise. Accessed Mar 17, 2019.

Schmitz KH, Ahmed RL, Troxel AB, et al. Weight lifting for women at risk for breast cancer-related lymphedema: A randomized trial. *JAMA*. 2010 Dec 22; 304 (24): 2699–705.

Tidhar D, Katz-Leurer M. Aqua lymphatic therapy in women who suffer from breast cancer treatment-related lymphedema: A randomized controlled study. *Support Care Cancer*. 2010 Mar; 18 (3): 383–92.

Tschentscher M, Niederseer D, Niebauer J. Health benefits of nordic walking: A systematic review. *Am J Prev Med*. 2013 Jan; 44 (1): 76–84.

Walter C. *Nordic Walking: The Complete Guide to Health, Fitness, and Fun*. Long Island City, NY: Hatherleigh Press, 2009.

Zhang X, Brown JC, Paskett ED, et al. Changes in arm tissue composition with slowly progressive weight-lifting among women with breast cancer-related lymphedema. *Breast Cancer Res Treat*. 2017 Jul; 164 (1): 79–88.

Zuther J. Yoga for lymphedema. *Lymphedema: Inform Yourself and Take Control*. Mar 2, 2017. Available at: www.lymphedemablog.com. Accessed Mar 17, 2019.

Chapter 9: Lymphatic Taping

Kase K, Stockheimer KR. *Kinesio Taping for Lymphoedema and Chronic Swelling*. Albuquerque, NM: Kinesio Taping Association, 2006.

Martins Jde C, Aguiar SS, Fabro EA, et al. Safety and tolerability of Kinesio Taping in patients with arm lymphedema: Medical device clinical study. *Support Care Cancer*. 2016 Mar; 24 (3): 1119–24.

Morris D, Jones D, Ryan H, et al. The clinical effects of Kinesio Tex taping: A systematic review. *Physiother Theory Pract*. 2013 May; 29 (4): 259–70.

Pekyavaş NÖ, Tunay VB, Akbayrak T, et al. Complex decongestive therapy and taping for patients with postmastectomy lymphedema: A randomized controlled study. *Eur J Oncol Nurs*. 2014 Dec; 18 (6): 585–90.

Taradaj J, Halski T, Rosinczuk J, et al. A. The influence of Kinesiology Taping on the volume of lymphoedema and manual dexterity of the upper limb in women after breast cancer treatment. *Eur J Cancer Care (Engl)*. 2016 Jul; 25 (4): 647–60.

Tsai HJ, Hung HC, Yang JL, et al. Could Kinesio tape replace the bandage in decongestive lymphatic therapy for breast-cancer-related lymphedema? A pilot study. *Support Care Cancer*. 2009 Nov; 17 (11): 1353–60.

Chapter 10: Body Weight and Lymphedema

Fletcher AM. *Thin for Life: 10 Keys to Success from People Who Have Lost Weight and Kept It Off*. New York: Rux Martin/Houghton Mifflin Harcourt, 2003.

Harvie MN, Pegington M, Mattson MP, et al. The effects of intermittent or continuous energy restriction on weight loss and metabolic disease risk markers: A randomized trial in young overweight women. *Int J Obes (Lond)*. 2011 May; 35 (5): 714–27.

Harvie M, Wright C, Pegington M, et al. The effect of intermittent energy and carbohydrate restriction v. daily energy restriction on weight loss and metabolic disease risk markers in overweight women. *Br J Nutr*. 2013 Oct; 110 (8): 1534–47.

Keith L; LE&RN Symposium Series. Diet and lifestyle for lymphatic disorders: Implementing a ketogenic diet. *Lymphatic Network*. Aug 28, 2017. Available at: https://lymphaticnetwork.org/symposium-series/diet-and-lifestyle-for-lymphatic-disorders-implementing-a-ketogenic-diet. Accessed Jul 2018.

Moro T, Tinsley G, Bianco A, et al. Effects of eight weeks of time-restricted feeding (16/8) on basal metabolism, maximal strength, body composition, inflammation, and cardiovascular risk factors in resistance-trained males. *J Transl Med*. 2016 Oct 13; 14 (1): 290.

Rothschild J, Hoddy KK, Jambazian P, et al. Time-restricted feeding and risk of metabolic disease: A review of human and animal studies. *Nutr Rev*. 2014 May; 72 (5): 308–18.

Shaw C, Mortimer P, Judd, PA. Randomized controlled trial comparing a low-fat diet with a weight-reduction diet in breast cancer-related lymphedema. *Cancer*. 2007 May 15; 109 (10): 1949–56.

Shaw C, Mortimer P, Judd PA. A randomized controlled trial of weight reduction as a treatment for breast cancer-related lymphedema. *Cancer*. 2007 Oct 15; 110 (8): 1868–74.

Studies Investigating the Risk Factors for Lymphedema in Cancer Patients

Ahmed RL, Schmitz KH, Prizment AE, et al. Risk factors for lymphedema in breast cancer survivors, the Iowa Women's Health Study. *Breast Cancer Res Treat*. 2011 Dec; 130 (3): 981–91.

Clark B, Sitzia J, Harlow W. Incidence and risk of arm oedema following treatment for breast cancer: A three-year follow-up study. *QJM*. 2005 May; 98 (5): 343–8.

DiSipio T, Rye S, Newman B, et al. Incidence of unilateral arm lymphoedema after breast cancer: A systematic review and meta-analysis. *Lancet Oncol*. 2013 May; 14 (6): 500–15.

Greene AK, Grant FD, Slavin SA. Lower-extremity lymphedema and elevated body-mass index. *N Engl J Med*. 2012 May 31; 366 (22): 2136–7.

Huang HP, Zhou JR, Zeng Q. Risk factors associated with lymphedema among postmenopausal breast cancer survivors after radical mastectomy and axillary dissection in China. *Breast Care (Basel)*. 2012 Dec; 7 (6): 461–4.

Jammallo LS, Miller CL, Singer M, et al. Impact of body mass index and weight fluctuation on lymphedema risk in patients treated for breast cancer. *Breast Cancer Res Treat.* 2013 Nov; 142 (1): 59–67.

Kilbreath SL, Refshauge KM, Beith JM, et al. Risk factors for lymphoedema in women with breast cancer: A large prospective cohort. *Breast.* 2016 Aug; 28: 29–36.

Mehrara BJ, Greene AK. Lymphedema and obesity: Is there a link? *Plast Reconstr Surg.* 2014 Jul; 134 (1): 154e–160e.

Rebegea L, Firescu D, Dumitru M, et al. The incidence and risk factors for occurrence of arm lymphedema after treatment of breast cancer. *Chirurgia (Bucur).* 2015 Jan–Feb; 110 (1): 33–7.

Ridner SH, Dietrich MS, Stewart BR, et al. Body mass index and breast cancer treatment-related lymphedema. *Support Care Cancer.* 2011 Jun; 19 (6): 853–7.

Treves N. An evaluation of the etiological factors of lymphedema following radical mastectomy: An analysis of 1,007 cases. *Cancer.* 1957 May–Jun; 10 (3): 444–59.

Chapter 11: Lymphatics and the Digestion of Dietary Fats

Advanced Renal Education Program. Chyloperitoneum. *Fresenius Medical Care.* Jun 2016. Available at: www.advancedrenaleducation.com/content/chyloperitoneum. Accessed Jul 2018.

Alexander JS, Ganta VC, Jordan PA, et al. Gastrointestinal lymphatics in health and disease. *Pathophysiology.* 2010 Sep; 17 (4): 315–35.

Blum KS, Karaman S, Proulx ST, et al. Chronic high-fat diet impairs collecting lymphatic vessel function in mice. *PLoS One.* 2014 Apr 8; 9 (4): e94713.

Chemistry Explained. Fats and fatty acids. *Chemistry Explained.* Available at: www.chemistryexplained.com/Di-Fa/Fats-and-Fatty-Acids.html. Accessed Jul 28, 2018.

Chempro Technovation. Top-notch technology in production of oils and fats. *Chempro Technovation.* Available at: www.chempro.in/fattyacid.htm. Accessed Jul 15, 2018.

Dixon JB. Lymphatic lipid transport: Sewer or subway? *Trends Endocrinol Metab.* 2010 Aug; 21 (8): 480–7.

Institute of Medicine. *Dietary Reference Intakes for Energy, Carbohydrate, Fiber, Fat, Fatty Acids, Cholesterol, Protein, and Amino Acids.* 2005. Washington, DC: National Academies Press. Available at: https://doi.org/10.17226/10490. Accessed Jul 19, 2018.

Mogensen K. Essential fatty acid deficiency. *Practical Gastroenterology.* Jun 2017; 164: 37–44.

National Institutes of Health. Primary intestinal lymphangiectasia. *U.S. Department of Health and Human Services.* Mar 2017. Available at: https://rarediseases.info.nih.gov/diseases/7873/primary-intestinal-lymphangiectasia. Accessed Jul 19, 2018.

Oliveira J, César TB. Influence of complex decongestive physical therapy associated with intake of medium-chain triglycerides for treating upper-limb lymphedema. *Rev Bras Fisioter.* 2008; 12 (1): 31–6.

Palmer S. The top fiber-rich foods list. *Today's Dietitian.* Jul 2008. Available at: www.todaysdietitian.com/newarchives/063008p28.shtml. Accessed Jul 19, 2018.

Shah N, Limketkai B. The use of medium-chain triglycerides in gastrointestinal disorders. *Practical Gastroenterology.* Feb 2017; 160: 20–8.

Soria P, Cuesta A, Romera H, et al. Dietary treatment of lymphedema by restriction of long-chain triglycerides. *Angiology.* 1994 Aug; 45 (8): 703–7.

Chapter 12: Reducing Chronic Inflammation

Alexander JS, Ganta VC, Jordan PA, et al. Gastrointestinal lymphatics in health and disease. *Pathophysiology.* 2010 Sep; 17 (4): 315–35.

Anft M. Understanding inflammation. *Johns Hopkins Health Review.* Spring/Summer 2016; 3 (1): 50–7.

Cavicchia PP, Steck SE, Hurley TG, et al. A new dietary inflammatory index predicts interval changes in serum high-sensitivity C-reactive protein. *J Nutr.* 2009 Dec; 139 (12): 2365–72.

Chrysohoou C, Panagiotakos DB, Pitsavos C, et al. Adherence to the Mediterranean diet attenuates inflammation and coagulation process in healthy adults the ATTICA study. *J Am Coll Cardiol.* 2004 Jul 7; 44 (1): 152–8.

Counzin-Frankel J. Inflammation bares a dark side. *Science.* 2010 Dec 17; 330 (6011): 1621.

Dietitians of Canada. Tips on how to avoid metabolic syndrome. *UnlockFood.ca.* Updated Jan 16, 2019. Available at: www.unlockfood.ca/en/Articles/Heart-Health/Tips-on-how-to-avoid-metabolic-syndrome.aspx. Accessed Mar 14, 2019.

DiNicolantonio JJ, O'Keefe JH. Importance of maintaining a low omega-6/omega-3 ratio for reducing inflammation. *Open Heart.* 2018 Nov 26; 5 (2): e000946.

Gotsis E, Anagnostis P, Mariolis A, et al. Health benefits of the Mediterranean diet: An update of research over the last 5 years. *Angiology.* 2015 Apr; 66 (4): 304–18.

Jones D, Min W. An overview of lymphatic vessels and their emerging role in cardiovascular disease. *J Cardiovasc Dis Res.* 2011 Jul; 2 (3): 141–52.

National Sunflower Association. High oleic sunflower oil. *National Sunflower Association.* Available at: www.sunflowernsa.com/oil/High-Oleic-Sunflower-Oil. Accessed Mar 7, 2019.

Pearson TA, Mensah GA, Alexander RW, et al. Markers of inflammation and cardiovascular disease: Application to clinical and public health practice; A statement for healthcare professionals from the Centers for Disease Control and Prevention and the American Heart Association. *Circulation.* 2003 Jan 28; 107 (3): 499–511.

Ricker MA, Haas WC. Anti-inflammatory diet in clinical practice; A review. *Nutr Clin Pract.* 2017 Jun; 32 (3): 318–25.

The Seven Countries Study. Available at: www.sevencountriesstudy.com. Accessed June 28, 2018.

Slavich G. Understanding inflammation, its regulation, and relevance for health: A top scientific and public priority. *Brain Behav Immun.* 2015 Mar; 45: 13–4.

Time. The secret killer: The surprising link between inflammation and heart attacks, cancer, Alzheimer's and other diseases; What you can do to fight it. Feb 23, 2004. *Time.* Available at: http://content.time.com/time/covers/0,16641,20040223,00.html. Accessed Mar 21, 2018.

Chapter 13: Fluid, Protein and Sodium

Canadian Food Inspection Agency. Sodium (salt) claims. Jan 15, 2019. *Government of Canada.* Available at: www.inspection.gc.ca/food/general-food-requirements-and-guidance/labelling/for-industry/nutrient-content/specific-claim-requirements/eng/1389907770176/1389907817577?chap=9. Accessed Mar 14, 2019.

Centers for Disease Control and Prevention. Get the facts: Sodium and the dietary guidelines. *Centers for Disease Control and Prevention.* Oct 2017. Available at: www.cdc.gov/salt/pdfs/sodium_dietary_guidelines.pdf. Accessed Mar 14, 2019.

Dietitians of Canada. Get the scoop on salt. *UnlockFood.ca.* Updated Jan 12, 2019. Available at: www.unlockfood.ca/en/Articles/Heart-Health/Get-the-Scoop-on-Salt.aspx. Accessed Mar 14, 2019.

Dietitians of Canada. How to prevent and treat the silent killer. *UnlockFood.ca*. Updated Jan 29, 2019. Available at: www.unlockfood.ca/en/Articles/Heart-Health/Hypertension-How-to-prevent-and-treat-the-silent.aspx. Accessed Mar 14, 2019.

Dietitians of Canada. Sodium sense. *Dietitians of Canada*. Jan 2015. Available at: www.dietitians.ca/Downloads/Factsheets/Sodium-Sense-factsheet-collection.aspx. Accessed Mar 14, 2019.

Food & Drug Administration. Use the nutrition facts label to reduce your intake of sodium in your diet. *U.S. Department of Health and Human Services*. Jun 12, 2018. Available at: www.fda.gov/food/resourcesforyou/consumers/ucm315393.htm. Accessed Mar 14, 2019.

Frank AP, Clegg DJ. Dietary guidelines for Americans: Eat less salt. *JAMA Network*. Aug 16, 2016. Available at: https://jamanetwork.com/journals/jama/fullarticle/2544642. Accessed Mar 17, 2019.

Frisoli TM, Schmieder RE, Grodzicki T, et al. Salt and hypertension: Is salt dietary reduction worth the effort? *Am J Med*. 2012 May; 125 (5): 433–9.

Health and Medicine Division. Dietary reference intakes tables and application: Electrolytes and water summary. *National Academies of Sciences Engineering Medicine*. Updated Jan 16, 2018. Available at: http://nationalacademies.org/HMD/Activities/Nutrition/SummaryDRIs/DRI-Tables.aspx. Accessed Jul 29, 2018.

Health Canada. Sodium in Canada. *Government of Canada*. Updated Mar 1, 2017. Available at: www.canada.ca/en/health-canada/services/food-nutrition/healthy-eating/sodium.html. Accessed Mar 14, 2019.

Institute of Medicine. *Dietary Reference Intakes for Water, Potassium, Sodium, Chloride, and Sulfate*. 2005. Washington, DC: National Academies Press. Available at: https://doi.org/10.17226/10925. Accessed Jul 17, 2018.

Mizuno R, Isshiki M, Ono N, et al. A high-salt diet differentially modulates mechanical activity of afferent and efferent collecting lymphatics in murine iliac lymph nodes. *Lymphat Res Biol*. 2015 Jun; 13 (2): 85–92.

National Health Service. Salt: The facts. *Department of Health and Social Care (DHSC)*. Updated Oct 2, 2018. Available at: www.nhs.uk/live-well/eat-well/salt-nutrition. Accessed Mar 14, 2019.

Office of Dietary Supplements. Dietary reference intakes (DRIs): Recommended dietary allowance and adequate intakes, total water and macronutrients. *National Institutes of Health*. 2011. Available at: www.ncbi.nlm.nih.gov/books/NBK56068/table/summarytables.t4/?report=objectonly. Accessed July 10, 2018.

Roberts HJ. Use of a low-sodium formula as an improved Karell diet, with emphasis upon the outpatient management of heart failure and lymphedema. *Am Heart J*. 1962 Jan; 65: 32–49.

World Health Organization. Salt reduction. *World Health Organization*. Jun 30, 2016. Available at: www.who.int/mediacentre/factsheets/fs393/en. Accessed Jul 14, 2018.

Zuther J. Diet and lymphedema. *Lymphedema: Inform Yourself and Take Control*. Mar 16, 2018. Available at: www.lymphedemablog.com/2018/03/16/diet-and-lymphedema. Accessed Mar 19, 2019.

Chapter 14: Supplements

Alwi I. Tips and tricks to make case report. *Acta Med Indones*. 2007 Apr–Jun; 39 (2): 96–8.

Budgell B. Guidelines to the writing of case studies. *J Can Chiropr Assoc*. 2008 Dec; 52 (4): 199–204.

Pfister C, Dawzcynski H, Schingale FJ. Sodium selenite and cancer related lymphedema: Biological and pharmacological effects. *J Trace Elem Med Biol*. 2016 Sep; 37: 111–6.

Poage EG, Rodrick JR, Wanchai A, et al. Exploring the usefulness of botanicals as an adjunctive treatment for lymphedema: A systematic search and review. *PM R*. 2015 Mar; 7 (3): 296–310.

Chapter 15: Meal Planning

Food and Nutrition Board. Dietary reference intakes (DRIs): Estimated average requirements. *National Academies of Sciences Engineering Medicine*. Updated Mar 5, 2019. Available at: http://nationalacademies.org/hmd/~/media/Files/Report%20Files/2019/DRI-Tables-2019/6_ DRIValues_Summary.pdf?la=en. Accessed Mar 21, 2019.

Johnson RK, Appel LJ, Brands M, et al, including American Heart Association Nutrition Committee of the Council on Nutrition, Physical Activity, and Metabolism and the Council on Epidemiology and Prevention. Dietary sugars intake and cardiovascular health: A scientific statement from the American Heart Association. *Circulation*. 2009 Sep 15; 120 (11): 1011–20.

Shaw C, Mortimer P, Judd, PA. Randomized controlled trial comparing a low-fat diet with a weight-reduction diet in breast cancer-related lymphedema. *Cancer*. 2007 May 15; 109 (10): 1949–56.

Shaw C, Mortimer P, Judd PA. A randomized controlled trial of weight reduction as a treatment for breast cancer-related lymphedema. *Cancer*. 2007 Oct 15; 110 (8): 1868–74.

Appendix 1: pH Levels of Skin Care Products

Ali SM, Yosipovitch G. Skin pH: From basic science to basic skin care. *Acta Derm Venereol*. 2013 May; 93 (3): 261–7.

Yosipovitch G, Maibach HI. Skin surface pH: A protective acid mantle. *Cosmet Toiletries*. 1996; 111: 101–2.

Appendix 3: Supplement Descriptions, Claims and Evidence

Badger C, Preston N, Seers K, et al. Benzo-pyrones for reducing and controlling lymphedema of the limbs. *Cochrane Database Syst Rev*. 2004; 2: CD003140.

Belcaro G, Dugall M, Hu S, et al. French oak wood (*Quercus robur*) extract (Robuvit) in primary lymphedema: A supplement, pilot, registry evaluation. *Int J Angiol*. 2015 Mar; 24 (1): 47–54.

Bruns F, Büntzel J, Mücke R, et al. Selenium in the treatment of head and neck lymphedema. *Med Princ Pract*. 2004 Jul–Aug; 13 (4): 185–90.

Cesarone MR, Belcaro G, Rohdewald P, et al. Prevention of edema in long flights with Pycnogenol. *Clin Appl Thromb Hemost*. 2005 Jul; 11 (3): 289–94.

Cluzan RV, Alliot F, Ghabboun S, et al. Treatment of secondary lymphedema of the upper limb with CYCLO 3 FORT. *Lymphology*. 1996 Mar; 29 (1): 29–35.

Cluzan RV, Pecking AP, Mathiex-Fortunet H, Léger Picherit E. Efficacy of BN165 (Ginkor Fort) in breast cancer related upper limb lymphedema: A preliminary study. *Lymphology*. 2004 Jun; 37 (2): 47–52.

Dennert G, Horneber M. Selenium for alleviating the side effects of chemotherapy, radiotherapy and surgery in cancer patients. *Cochrane Database Syst Rev*. 2006 Jul 19; 3: CD005037.

Dini D, Bianchini M, Massa T, et al. Treatment of upper limb lymphedema after mastectomy with escine and lev-thyroxine. [Article in Italian.] *Minerva Med*. 1981 Sep 22; 72 (35): 2319–22.

Farinola N, Piller N. Pharmacogenoimics: Its role in re-establishing coumarin as treatment for lymphedema. *Lymphat Res Biol*. 2005 Summer; 3 (2): 81–6.

Gothard L, Cornes P, Earl J, et al. Double-blind placebo-controlled randomized trial of vitamin E and pentoxifylline in patients with chronic arm lymphoedema and fibrosis after surgery and radiotherapy for breast cancer. *Radiother Oncol*. 2004 Nov; 73 (2): 133–9.

Huston P. Horse chestnut seed extract for lymphedema. Unpublished research. Available at https://clinicaltrials.gov/ct2/show/NCT00213928?term=horse+chestnut&cond=Lymphedema&rank=1. Personal correspondence, July 29, 2018.

Huston P. Pycnogenol for the treatment of lymphedema. Unpublished research. Available at https://clinicaltrials.gov/ct2/show/NCT00214032?term=pine+bark&rank=7. Personal correspondence, June 29, 2018.

Kasseroller R. Sodium selenite as prophylaxis against erysipelas in secondary lymphedema. *Anticancer Res*. 1998 May–Jun; 18 (3C): 2227–30.

Kasseroller RG, Schrauzer GN. Treatment of secondary lymphedema of the arm with physical decongestive therapy and sodium selenite: A review. *Am J Ther*. 2000 Aug; 7 (4): 273–9.

Korpan MI, Fialka V. Wobezyme and diuretic therapy in lymphedema after breast operation. [Article in German.] *Wien Med Wochenschr*. 1996; 146 (4): 67–72; discussion 74.

Loprinzi CL, Kugler JW, Sloan JA, et al. Lack of effect of coumarin in women with lymphedema after treatment for breast cancer. *N Engl J Med*. 1999 Feb 4; 340 (5): 346–50.

Micke O, Bruns F, Mücke R, et al. Selenium in the treatment of radiation-associated secondary lymphedema. *Int J Radiat Oncol Biol Phys*. 2003 May 1; 56 (1): 40–9.

Natural Medicines Database. *Therapeutic Research Center*. Available at: https://naturalmedicines.therapeuticresearch.com. Accessed Mar 2018.

Pecking A. Medical treatment of lymphedema with benzopyrones: Experimental basis and applications. [Article in French.] *J Mal Vasc*. 1990; 15 (2): 157–8.

Pecking AP. Evaluation by lymphoscintigraphy of the effect of a micronized flavonoid fraction (Daflon 500 mg) in the treatment of upper limb lymphedema. *Int Angiol*. 1995 Sep; 14 (3 Suppl 1): 39–43.

Pecking AP, Février B, Wargon C, et al. Efficacy of Daflon 500 mg in the treatment of lymphedema (secondary to conventional therapy of breast cancer). *Angiology*. 1997 Jan; 48 (1): 93–8.

Pfister C, Dawzcynski H, Schingale FJ. Sodium selenite and cancer related lymphedema: Biological and pharmacological effects. *J Trace Elem Med Biol*. 2016 Sep; 37: 111–6.

Pittler MH, Ernst E. Horse chestnut seed extract for chronic venous insufficiency. *Cochrane Database Syst Rev*. 2012 Nov 14; 11: CD003230.

Priya MD, Elenjikkal S. Traditional and modern use of Indian madder (*Rubia cordifolia* L.): An overview. *Int J Pharm Sci Rev Res*. 2014 Jan 27: 154–64.

Scheepers L. Galium aparine proving report. *Homeopathic Centre Antwerp*. Dec 2006. Available at: www.provings.info/pruefungen.html/galium%20aparine%20scheepers%20en.pdf?pruefung=galium%20aparine%20scheepers%20en.pdf. Accessed July 24, 2018

Underland V, Saeterdal I, Nilsen ES. Cochrane summary of findings: Horse chestnut for chronic venous insufficiency. *Glob Adv Health Med*. 2012 Mar; 1 (1): 122–3.

Vettorello G, Cerreta G, Derwish A, et al. Contribution of a combination of alpha and beta benzopyrones, flavonoids, and natural terpenes in the treatment of lymphedema of the lower limbs at the 2d stage of the surgical classification. [Article in Italian.] *Minerva Cardioangiol*. 1996 Sep; 44 (9): 447–55.

Wollina U, Abdel-Naser MB, Mani R. A review of the microcirculation in skin in patients with chronic venous insufficiency: The problem and the evidence available for therapeutic options. *Int J Low Extrem Wounds*. 2006 Sep; 5 (3): 169–80.

Zimmerman T, Leonhardt H, Kersting S, et al. Reduction of postoperative lymphedema after oral tumor surgery with sodium selenite. *Biol Trace Elem Res*. 2005 Sep; 106 (3): 193–203.

Before and After Treatment

1. The person in the first pair of photos had secondary lymphedema in his left arm for several months before beginning treatment, which consisted of skin care, MLD, exercises and compression bandaging three times per week. The "after" photo was taken 4 weeks after treatment began. Further reductions were made before he was fitted for compression garments.

2. The person in the second pair of photos had had secondary lymphedema in her left arm for many years. It had been stable, but she had recently experienced a flare-up of her swelling. The "after" photo was taken 2 weeks after the initiation of treatment (as described above). Further reductions were made before she was fitted for compression garments.

3. The person in the third pair of photos had primary leg lymphedema. Their right leg was prone to cellulitis infections, which resulted in significantly more swelling on that side. The "after" photo was taken 6 weeks after the initiation of treatment (as described above).

1. Arm Lymphedema

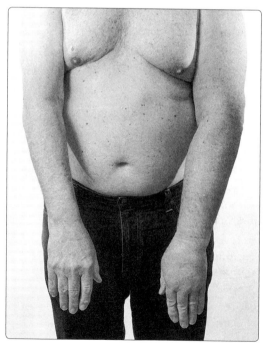

BEFORE

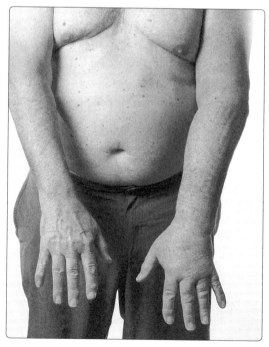

AFTER

2. Arm Lymphedema

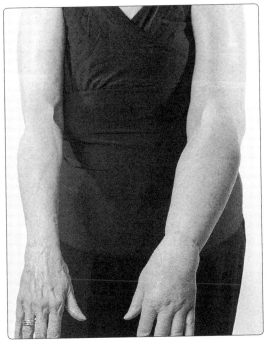 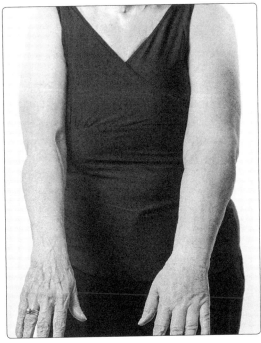

BEFORE   *AFTER*

3. Leg Lymphedema

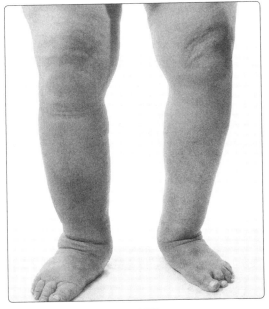 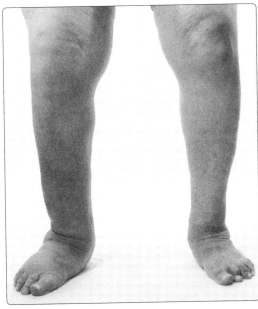

BEFORE   *AFTER*

Living with Lymphedema: Personal Stories

Story #1

When I had my second surgery for melanoma, I was informed that it would likely result in leg lymphedema. Although surgery and recovery were uneventful, weeks later, when the stitches were removed, the surgical site became infected and secondary leg lymphedema followed.

While learning to live with lymphedema required a significant adjustment, the most important factor has been education, for myself and my family. I've had to learn how to best manage my leg without it being a limitation, and I've had to educate my family about this condition.

I now know that it's especially beneficial to follow a healthy, balanced diet and to maintain regular exercise while keeping my weight stable. Happily, I am able to continue enjoying the same level of physical activity as always: walking, hiking, bike riding, spinning, yoga, dancing, Pilates, as well as cardio and weight workouts at the gym.

I have learned that to effectively manage lymphedema, it is essential to find a trusted garment fitter to advise you on the best possible compression wear for your needs, and to take good care of your compression wear, ideally replacing garments every 4 months.

I have learned that finding a competent physiotherapist with expertise in MLD, to provide regular treatment, is imperative to keep the affected limb stable and healthy. I have also found it to be extremely beneficial to learn MLD techniques in order to maintain daily self-care, which is part of my routine two or three times per day, depending on my level of activity.

I am sharing my experience in the hope that it will help others who find themselves having to adjust to the new normal of living with lymphedema.

Story #2

I don't know if my experience with lymphedema is common or unique. However, there is no question in my mind that its diagnosis and treatment were unnecessarily delayed.

Lymphedema has a number of triggers. Mine was trauma caused by a broken ankle followed immediately by deep vein thrombosis (a blood clot). My orthopedist informed me that my healing ankle would remain swollen for quite a while. I took him at his word. Many months went by, and it was still swollen. A year, two years, three years passed. By that time, the swelling had spread from my ankle to my leg. My general practitioner kept monitoring it and eventually prescribed compression socks, off the rack. No improvement.

My GP then sent me to a vascular surgeon who, after some tests, wanted to operate. I went for a second opinion at a major hospital's vascular department. That's the first time I heard the term "lymphedema," along with a strong caution against surgery. The first real treatment for my lymphedema began. My leg was wrapped and monitored. Finally, after a number of weeks, the swelling was down to normal and all was good. Or so I thought. Although I now had compression socks, I did not wear them religiously. No one gave me ongoing guidance, and there was no long-term monitoring or treatment. The consensus seemed to be that the wraps had done their work, and we were done. Except that we weren't. The swelling returned!

Purely by happenstance, while I was on a hunt to find shoes that would fit my swollen foot, a specialty shoe maven informed me that, with lymphedema, there is a need for ongoing treatment and monitoring. She referred me to a center with the knowledge and expertise my condition required. There, I was evaluated, diagnosed, wrapped and educated. Specially trained physiotherapists massaged and drained the lymphatic fluids from my system. I was finally on my way to proper and full control of my lymphedema.

My only question: Why did it take more than 5 years to get to this point? And I'm one of the fortunate ones!

Story #3

I have been managing lymphedema for almost 5 years. After a mastectomy and removal of about 34 lymph nodes, followed by chemo and radiation, I developed lymphedema in my right arm, side and back. The lymphedema nurse at the hospital measured the circumference of my arm over a period of 6 months and noticed it was getting larger. I was measured for compression sleeves and gauntlets, which would keep the swelling down during the day. At first I felt quite upset about needing to wear these uncomfortable garments, but now I feel they are my best friends! I also wear a compression vest and underwear. All of these items (I call them my armor) help to keep the swelling under control. I can exercise and perform everyday activities because the garments give me support.

I go to a very knowledgeable physiotherapist who specializes in lymphedema and manual lymphatic drainage. When she finishes treating me, my arm is smaller and feels great! She has taught me how to do self-MLD, and I do it at least once or twice a day, before bed or first thing in the morning. At first this was challenging because I had to use my left hand to treat my right arm and I am right-handed. However, now it is quite easy, as I have developed dexterity and strength in my left arm and hand. The self-MLD combined with the compression garments keep me pretty comfortable.

I took a special yoga course for lymphedema and learned to do breathing exercises that help push the lymphatic fluid around. Whenever I think of it, even in the car, I do those exercises. They do help. I also try to avoid stress, challenging though it may be. I find that prolonged stress exacerbates the swelling. Too much sitting also makes it worse. When I travel, I wear a compression glove on the plane because the air pressure when flying is less than on the ground. I get an aisle seat and walk around a lot too.

Swimming is a great activity because the hydrostatic pressure from the water acts like compression. I try to get into a pool whenever I can and stay submerged up to my neck to get the maximum benefit.

I limit salt, drink water and try to eat small, healthy meals, especially at dinner. I usually have a lot of energy, and for that I am very grateful. It has all become my new normal!

Acknowledgments

From Ann & Jean

We are very grateful for the great team at Robert Rose, including Bob Dees, Kelly Glover and Megan Brush; your expertise and guidance were exactly what we needed and we appreciate your dedication to our book. Our amazing editors Sue Sumeraj, Kelly Jones and Jennifer MacKenzie did a great job in refining and organizing our text and recipes and creating a cohesive project; we especially appreciate Kelly's willingness to jump in at the eleventh hour to help us create a book that we are so proud of. To the team at PageWave Graphics, Joseph Gisini, Kevin Cockburn and Daniella Zanchetta, who provided excellent guidance around photography and images and made our book beautiful. Thank you to Colleen Wood, who did preliminary sketches for the book that helped shape our decisions on final images we would need to support our text.

To our focus group, thank you for offering the wisdom and guidance about what it is like to live with lymphedema and assisting our readers in a way that neither of us can. To our models, we appreciate and acknowledge your brave willingness to be photographed to help others.

To Dr. Ewa Szumacher, who took time away from her busy practice as a radiation oncologist to read our manuscript and provide a forward. We would also like to thank Sally Keefe Cohen, a most excellent literary consultant who helped us understand the business side of creating this book. Thank you to Ted Overton for filming the videos that will go live on our website, www. MarkhamLymphaticCentre.com, and will provide a valuable support to our book. To all of our readers, we thank you for your trust in us by choosing this book to guide you with your lymphedema and especially to those who take the extra step to write reviews for us on Amazon and other sites, to share on social media and to recommend to others who may benefit from our book. Thank you for helping us get the word out.

From Ann

Writing this book was harder than I thought it would be, but it was an amazing and rewarding experience. Teaching clients to manage lymphedema is something I do every single day, and to write a book on the topic was a natural extension of my everyday practice.

The thousands of people whom I have had the privilege to serve over the past 10 years were my inspiration for this project. You graciously shared your stories with me and allowed me to help you manage your lymphedema; I want to say thank you for being the genesis and foundation for this project. It is from you that my strength and passion to improve recognition and treatment for this condition are derived.

There are some individuals whom I would like to mention. Thank you to Tania Oblijubek for helping me with the research component of this project and for proofreading the original manuscript for its medical soundness.

Thank you to Jan McFarland, who trained me 10 years ago in integrated lymph drainage at Toronto Lymphocare. You taught me to work holistically with my patients through the mind-body-and-spirit connection and to trust my hands. You encouraged me to carry on with this work and were always there to provide support.

A special thank-you to the team of amazing certified lymphedema therapists at Markham Lymphatic Centre, Pooja Arora, Anne Marie Chlorakos and Kaushika Logeswaran, who work tirelessly with me each day to make the lives of our patients better. Your support of our shared vision to teach self-management and increase awareness about lymphedema is so important to me. This book is our combined achievement! I also want to acknowledge our great administration staff, Melody Field and Susan Howitt, who always manage to find the perfect words to comfort our clients and reassure them that they will receive the care and guidance they need.

To Jean, who took a chance two years ago by joining the team at Markham Lymphatic Centre and who digs through the research to determine how nutrition can complement the work that we do, you are truly a kind, caring and brilliant person who will help me move lymphedema management strategies to the next level.

Thank you to our photography coach, Rob Davidson, for teaching me how to take the best photos in a tight space with limited time. The patience you provided for my early photography trials and tribulations will not be forgotten.

To my family for all your support and encouragement over the years: you have all taught me the importance of hard work, dedication and perseverance. To my loving husband, Bernie, who 10 years ago encouraged me to follow my passion and start my own practice treating lymphedema, you have been a rock throughout the entire 10 years and have given me so many helpful suggestions. Thank you for helping me with all the technical details of this book.

To my children, thank you for believing your mom could write this book and accepting that I needed time to do it. Your patience throughout the writing process gave me the strength to power through it all. I love that you recognize that your mom helps and teaches people how to deal with lymphedema.

Ann Di Menna, PT, CDT
www.markhamlymphaticcentre.com

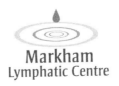

> "If you don't like something, change it. If you can't change it, change your attitude."
>
> — *Maya Angelou*

From Jean

I loved writing this book. I loved it because I love researching, writing and creating and because I have a strong belief that this book will make a difference for people with lymphedema. That inner belief kept me going, knowing that there are people out there who I can help. This book will help me reach them in a way that private one-on-one counselling never could. Writing a book is both an art and a science. When it comes to science, there are many who helped research this book whom I would like to acknowledge: Stella Aslibekyan, Linda Kelemen and Claire LaMantia. You set aside your own work to help me find the research I needed and you kept the project moving forward, enabling me to produce a trustworthy, evidence-based work. For my friends and dietitian colleagues Pam Osborne and Marilyn Mori, who provided a detailed review and editing of my section, including a review of all the research that I cited, what an amazing help you both were to me and the book, helping to ensure that the recommendations that I made were based on science, thereby contributing to the manuscript's being turned into a resource for nutrition professionals around the world through PEN (Practice-Based Evidence in Nutrition).

I would like to thank all the recipe contributors — the home economists, registered dietitians and recipe developers — who allowed me to select from their works the recipes that meet the unique needs of people with lymphedema. Thanks also to Monica Reinagel, creator of the IF Tracker app, with her dedication to quantifying inflammatory and anti-inflammatory foods, which has provided our readers with a tool to help them manage their lymphedema. To Nesreen Hajjar, who is my partner on the Cancer Risk Reduction Guide (www.CancerRiskReductionGuide.com) and who created amazing images for this book that help people with lymphedema understand digestion and how what they eat can affect their lymphedema, your images are worth more than a thousand words.

Last, I want to acknowledge my kids, who are my cheerleaders and who like to tell random strangers, "Our mom's a registered dietitian" and "My mom wrote a book that helps people." Your pride in me and my work makes me want to be the best dietitian and author I can be and help as many people with lymphedema as I can. Thank you for your enthusiasm and support of my work.

Jean LaMantia, RD
Dietitian, Survivor, Speaker
www.jeanlamantia.com
www.CancerRiskReductionGuide.com

CANCER RISK REDUCTION GUIDE

Jean LaMantia

Dietitian | Survivor | Speaker

Contributing Authors

Nesreen Al Hajjar
A recipe by this contributor is found on page 199.

Johanna Burkhard
500 Best Comfort Food Recipes
A recipe from this book is found on page 205.

Dietitians of Canada
Cook!
Recipes from this book are found on pages 196, 206, 219, 220 and 228.

Dietitians of Canada
Cook Great Food
Recipes from this book are found on pages 186, 201, 232 and 236.

Dietitians of Canada
Great Food Fast
Recipes from this book are found on pages 192, 195, 224, 234 and 235.

Dietitians of Canada
Simply Great Food
Recipes from this book are found on pages 207, 210, 212, 214, 217, 218, 221, 222, 223 and 226.

Judith Finlayson
The Complete Gluten-Free Whole Grains Cookbook
A recipe from this book is found on page 227.

Judith Finlayson
The Healthy Slow Cooker
Recipes from this book are found on pages 204 and 211.

Judith Finlayson
The Vegetarian Slow Cooker
A recipe from this book is found on page 237.

Marilyn Haugen
175 Best Superfood Blender Recipes Using Your Nutribullet®
Recipes from this book are found on pages 209, 215, 230, 238 and 239.

Rose Reisman
Rose Reisman Brings Home Light Cooking
Recipes from this book are found on pages 188, 189, 193, 194, 198 and 200.

Rose Reisman
Rose Reisman's Enlightened Home Cooking
A recipe from this book is found on page 197.

Rose Reisman
Rose Reisman's Light Vegetarian Cooking
A recipe from this book is found on page 233.

The recipes on pages 187, 190, 191, 202, 208, 216, 225, 231 and 240 were written by Jean LaMantia and are being published for the first time in this book.

Image Credits

Ann DiMenna: pages 22, 26, 45, 54–59, 65–73, 78, 84, 86, 97–106, 120–24 and 270–71.

BSN Medical — An Essity Company: page 89 (left). Used with permission.

DepositPhotos.com: pages 16 and 19.

Juzo Canada Ltd.: pages 18, 23 and 129. Used with permission.

Nesreen Al Hajjar: pages 144 and 166.

Sigvaris Group Canada: page 89 (right). Used with permission.

Library and Archives Canada Cataloguing in Publication

Title: The complete lymphedema management and nutrition guide : empowering strategies, supporting recipes
    & therapeutic exercises / Jean LaMantia, RD and Ann DiMenna, PT, CDT ; with foreword by Ewa Szumacher, MD,
    FRCP(C), MEd.
Names: LaMantia, Jean, author. I DiMenna, Ann, author. I Szumacher, Ewa, writer of foreword.
Description: Includes index.
Identifiers: Canadiana 20190094982 I ISBN 9780778806271 (softcover)
Subjects: LCSH: Lymphedema—Diet therapy—Popular works. I LCSH: Lymphedema—Exercise therapy—Popular
    works. I LCSH: Lymphedema—Prevention—Popular works. I LCSH: Lymphedema—Nutritional aspects—
    Popular works. I LCSH: Lymphedema—Diet therapy—Recipes.
Classification: LCC RC646.3 .L36 2019 I DDC 616.4/206—dc23

Index

lymph nodes, 17, 21
    removal of, 31–32, 36
lymphoscintigraphy, 27, 93

M

madder, 250
manual lymphatic drainage (MLD),
    48–59
    for arms, 55–56
    cautions, 50, 53
    effects, 49, 50–52
    for legs, 57–59
    vs. massage, 49
    for neck, 54–55
    research on, 50–52
    of self, 52–59
marshmallow root, 250
massage, 49
MCT oil, 146, 154, 162. *See also*
    medium-chain triglycerides
meals. *See also* diet; eating
    balancing, 130–32
    1500-calorie, 179, 180
    1800-calorie, 179, 181
    2100-calorie, 179, 182
    limits for, 178
    and lymphatic volume, 17
    planning, 177–82
    recording, 135
Mediterranean diet, 160–61
medium-chain triglycerides, 151–52.
    See also MCT oil
metabolic syndrome, 159
MLD. *See* manual lymphatic
    drainage
moisturizers, 46, 241, 243
mouth, 142–43
MRI (magnetic resonance imaging),
    27
muscle pump, 96
mushrooms, 251
    Barley with Mushrooms and
        Caramelized Onions, 228
    Broccoli and Mushroom Stir-Fry
        with Tofu, 216

Caramelized Onion and Roasted
    Mushroom Soup, 206
Cranberry Chicken Chili, 212
Lentils Bolognese, 214
Warm Mushroom and Snow Pea
    Salad, 193

N

n-acetyl cysteine, 250
nail infections, 46
near-infrared fluorescence imaging, 27
neck
    compression garments, 88–89
    lymphatic taping, 121
    MLD, 54–55
needle punctures, 34
Nordic pole walking, 110–11
nuts
    Beet Salad with Goat Cheese
        and Toasted Walnuts, 190
    Lemon Pesto Sauce, 232
    Warm Chicken Salad with
        Orange Dressing, 200

O

obesity, 36, 127. *See also* body weight;
    weight loss
oils, 149–52
    fatty acids in, 150–52, 160, 161
    to limit, 160, 161
    MCT, 146, 154, 162
    types, 151
oleic acid, 160
onions
    Barley with Mushrooms and
        Caramelized Onions, 228
    Broccoli and Mushroom Stir-Fry
        with Tofu, 216
    Caramelized Onion and Roasted
        Mushroom Soup, 206
    Stir-Fried Chinese Greens, 226
oranges and orange juice
    Carrot, Mango, Citrus and Ginger
        Smoothie with Hemp Seeds, 239